BLOOD TYPE O DIET COOKBOOK

Healthy Flavorful Recipes Tailored to Your Type O for Optimal Health and Wellness

LENA R. FOSTER

Blood Type O Diet Cookbook

Table of Contents

INTRODUCTION..**8**
CHAPTER 1: UNDERSTANDING BLOOD TYPE O........**10**
  BENEFITS OF FOLLOWING BLOOD TYPE O DIET.12
  FOODS TO EAT AND FOODS TO AVOID.................13
  SHOPPING LISTS FOR BLOOD TYPE O.................14
  TIPS FOR A SUCCESSFUL BLOOD TYPE O DIET..17
CHAPTER 2: 30-DAY MEAL PLAN.........................**18**
CHAPTER 3: BREAKFAST.................................**28**
  Omelet with Spinach and Turkey............................28
  Greek Yogurt Parfait with Berries...........................29
  Sweet Potato and Turkey Hash..............................30
  Quinoa Breakfast Bowl..31
  Egg and Spinach Breakfast Wrap..........................32
  Salmon and Avocado Toast....................................33
  Banana Almond Butter Smoothie Bowl...................34
  Turkey and Sweet Potato Breakfast Hash.............35
  Spinach and Mushroom Breakfast Quesadilla.........36
  Pumpkin Spice Chia Pudding Parfait.....................37
  Egg and Vegetable Breakfast Muffins....................39
  Apple Cinnamon Quinoa Breakfast Bowl................40
  Turkey and Vegetable Breakfast Burrito................41
  Blueberry Almond Breakfast Quinoa......................42
  Mushroom and Spinach Breakfast Frittata.............43
CHAPTER 4: LUNCH.......................................**46**
  Grilled Chicken and Vegetable Salad.....................46
  Salmon and Quinoa Bowl with Lemon-Dill Dressing.. 47

Turkey and Avocado Wrap with Greens....................49
Eggplant and Chickpea Salad Bowl...........................50
Lentil and Vegetable Stuffed Bell Peppers..................52
Shrimp and Zucchini Noodle Stir-Fry.........................53
Chicken and Broccoli Quinoa Bowl...........................54
Tuna and Avocado Lettuce Wraps...........................55
Beef and Vegetable Stir-Fry with Cauliflower Rice.....57
Turkey and Sweet Potato Hash................................58
Salmon and Asparagus Foil Packets.........................59
Chicken and Kale Caesar Salad...............................61
Egg and Turkey Spinach Wrap................................62
Miso-Ginger Salmon Bowl.....................................63
Quinoa and Black Bean Stuffed Peppers..................64
CHAPTER 5: SNACKS AND DESSERTS......................66
Turkey and Veggie Roll-Ups................................. 66
Apple and Almond Butter Slices............................. 67
Spicy Edamame...68
Cucumber and Smoked Salmon Bites.......................69
Almond Butter Banana Bites.................................70
Avocado and Tomato Salsa.................................. 71
Roasted Red Pepper Hummus Stuffed Mini Bell
Peppers.. 72
Crispy Chickpea and Rosemary Popcorn Mix............ 73
Baked Zucchini Chips...74
Cajun Roasted Nuts..75
Mango and Chili Lime Salsa with Jicama Slices.........76
Dark Chocolate-Dipped Strawberries with Almonds...77
Coconut Chia Pudding with Fresh Berries..................78
Frozen Banana and Almond Butter Bites.................. 79
Pomegranate and Mint Sorbet...............................80

Baked Cinnamon Apple Slices.................................. 81

Mint Chocolate Avocado Mousse............................. 82

CHAPTER 6: DINNER... 84

Grilled Lemon Garlic Chicken with Roasted Vegetables 84

Spiced Turkey and Quinoa Stuffed Bell Peppers........86

Turkey and Vegetable Stir-Fry with Ginger-Soy Sauce.. 88

Lemon Herb Grilled Chicken Salad............................ 90

Beef and Broccoli Stir-Fry with Garlic-Ginger Sauce.. 92

Grilled Shrimp and Zucchini Skewers with Lemon-Herb Marinade... 93

Sweet Potato and Turkey Chili.................................95

Lemon Herb Baked Cod with Roasted Brussels Sprouts..96

Chicken and Vegetable Stir-Fry with Cashew Nuts.... 98

Turkey and Spinach Stuffed Bell Peppers................ 100

Sesame Ginger Chicken Stir-Fry with Vegetables.... 101

Lemon Garlic Shrimp with Quinoa and Roasted Vegetables.. 103

Balsamic Glazed Chicken with Roasted Brussels Sprouts and Butternut Squash................................105

Miso-Glazed Salmon with Stir-Fried Bok Choy and Shiitake Mushrooms.. 106

Lemon Herb Grilled Chicken with Asparagus........... 108

Turkey and Vegetable Skillet with Cauliflower Rice.. 110

Spicy Shrimp and Broccoli Stir-Fry with Quinoa........111

Salmon and Avocado Salad with Citrus Vinaigrette.. 113

CHAPTER 7: NOURISHING SOUPS AND STEWS...... 116

Chicken and Vegetable Soup with Turmeric............. 116

Spicy Lentil and Spinach Soup.............................. 118

Beef and Sweet Potato Stew..................................... 119

Mushroom and Kale Miso Soup...............................120

Cabbage and Sausage Soup...................................122

Chickpea and Vegetable Stew with Turmeric.......... 123

Lentil and Turkey Sausage Soup.............................125

Quinoa and Vegetable Stew..................................... 126

Shrimp and Vegetable Coconut Soup......................127

Turkey and Butternut Squash Stew.......................... 129

Chicken and Mushroom Barley Stew........................130

Spicy Lentil and Kale Soup..................................... 132

Beef and Sweet Potato Stew................................... 133

CHAPTER 8: FISH AND POULTRY DISHES.............. 136

Baked Lemon Herb Salmon....................................136

Grilled Herb Chicken Breast with Lemon................. 137

Rosemary Lemon Chicken Skewers........................138

Garlic Ginger Turkey Stir-Fry.................................. 140

Baked Dijon Herb Tilapia.. 141

Lemon Garlic Butter Salmon Packets......................142

Lemon Herb Chicken Thighs................................... 144

Balsamic Honey Glazed Chicken Breasts................ 145

Coconut Lime Baked Cod....................................... 146

Herb-Crusted Baked Salmon.................................. 147

Mango Chipotle Grilled Chicken.............................. 148

Pesto Baked Trout... 150

CHAPTER 9: VEGETABLE DISHES............................ 152

Roasted Asparagus with Lemon and Parmesan...... 152

Mushroom and Spinach Sauté with Garlic...............153

Grilled Eggplant with Tahini Dressing...................... 154

Sweet Potato and Kale Hash...................................155

Zesty Broccoli and Bell Pepper Stir-Fry....................156

Spaghetti Squash Primavera....................158

Cauliflower and Chickpea Curry....................159

Stir-Fried Asparagus with Almonds....................161

Turmeric Roasted Carrots....................162

CHAPTER 10: SMOOTHIES....................164

Berry Green Smoothie....................164

Tropical Green Smoothie....................165

Citrus Berry Blast Smoothie....................166

Peachy Green Energizer Smoothie....................167

Minty Blueberry Bliss Smoothie....................168

Tangy Mango Turmeric Smoothie....................169

Berry Beet Burst Smoothie....................170

Pineapple Ginger Zing Smoothie....................171

Citrus Minty Greens Smoothie....................172

Apple Cinnamon Crunch Smoothie....................173

Mango Avocado Bliss Smoothie....................174

CONCLUSION....................176

TYPE O DIET WEEKLY MEAL PLANNER....................178

INTRODUCTION

Clara, a vivacious lady with blood type O, set out on a path to adopt a healthier lifestyle. Intrigued by the notion of tailored nutrition, she came upon a Blood Type O Diet Cookbook that claimed to improve her health.

Clara was taken through a series of meals designed precisely to her blood type by the cookbook. She experimented with tasty meals high in lean proteins such as chicken and fish, as well as a variety of vegetables and fruits. Clara enjoyed experimenting with new cuisines while adhering to her blood type's dietary requirements.

Clara observed an increase in her energy and general vigor after adopting the Blood Type O diet. Her mornings began with hearty breakfasts of eggs and leafy greens, which gave her energy throughout the day. Clara's lunches and dinners were bright arrays of stir-fried veggies, grilled chicken, and fish, ensuring that her meals were both satisfying and healthy.

Clara supplemented her meals with helpful activities according to her blood type. Regular bouts of strenuous exercises and relaxing yoga practices were part of her daily routine, contributing to a holistic approach to health.

Clara's friends and family noticed the wonderful change in her lifestyle. Inspired by her passion, they, too, started researching tailored diet based on their blood type. They developed a supportive group by sharing recipes, fitness advice, and the joys of living a healthy lifestyle.

In Clara's quest to embrace healthy living with her Blood Type O, the cookbook served as more than just a guide, offering up a world of culinary possibilities that enabled her to live with vigor and enjoyment.

Welcome to this gastronomic experience designed just for those with blood type O. In this Blood Type O Diet Cookbook, we go on a journey to discover the secrets of tailored nutrition, delving into a vivid tapestry of tastes and ingredients that cater to the specific demands of blood type O persons.

CHAPTER 1: UNDERSTANDING BLOOD TYPE O

Blood Type O is one of four major blood types, distinguished by the presence or lack of certain antigens on the surface of red blood cells.

Here are some important components of knowing Blood Type O:

1. Universal Donor: Blood Type O is known as the "universal donor" because people with this blood type may give blood to people of all blood types. This is due to the lack of A and B antigens on their red blood cells.

2. Genetic Inheritance: Blood type is inherited from parents. A person with Blood Type O might have gotten the O gene from both parents, resulting in Blood Type O, or an O gene from one parent and an A or B gene from the other, resulting in Blood Type A or B.

3. Rh Factor: The presence or absence of the Rh factor determines whether blood Type O is positive (+) or negative (-). The Rh factor is another antigen found on the surface of red blood cells.

4. Dietary Recommendations: The Blood Type O Diet indicates that those with Blood Type O may benefit from certain dietary choices. This involves prioritizing lean meats, certain fruits and vegetables, and eliminating certain grains and dairy.

5. Health Considerations: While some individuals benefit from following the Blood Type O Diet, it is important to emphasize that scientific data showing a clear relationship between blood type and dietary demands is limited. Individual health and nutritional needs differ, and other variables influence total well-being.

6. Compatibility in Blood Transfusions: Blood Type O negative is very useful in emergencies since it may be safely transfused into anyone with any blood type without triggering a response. Blood Type O positive is also a universal donor for Rh-positive recipients.

Understanding your blood type is essential for medical procedures like blood transfusions, organ transplants and also useful for investigating nutritional approaches.

BENEFITS OF FOLLOWING BLOOD TYPE O DIET

The Blood Type O Diet is thought to have numerous possible benefits:

1. Weight Control: The diet promotes lean proteins and precise dietary selections, which may assist in weight control by boosting metabolism and muscle mass.

2. Digestive Health: Customized meal choices may encourage improved digestion for those with blood type O, lowering the risk of digestive problems.

3. Energy Levels: A focus on protein-rich diets and healthy carbs may help to maintain energy levels throughout the day.

4. Immune System Support: A diet aligned with blood type O guidelines may help promote a strong immune system by consuming nutrient-dense foods.

5. Reduced Inflammation: Some people report a decrease in inflammation-related difficulties after avoiding foods that may be incompatible with their blood type.

6. Improved Mental Clarity: A well-balanced diet rich in nutrient-dense foods may benefit cognitive function and clarity.

7. Optimized Metabolism: The emphasis on certain meals is intended to correspond with the metabolic features associated with blood type O, possibly optimizing metabolic processes.

8. Better Blood Circulation: The diet emphasizes foods that may benefit cardiovascular health, hence improving blood circulation and heart health.

FOODS TO EAT AND FOODS TO AVOID

Foods to Eat for Blood Type O Diet

1. Lean Protein: Include lean meats such as beef, lamb, and chicken. Fish, especially those high in omega-3 fatty acids like salmon and mackerel, are also healthy.

2. Vegetables: Focus on kale, spinach, broccoli, and Brussels sprouts. These give important nutrients without negatively impacting blood type O.

3. Fruits: Choose berries, cherries, and plums. These fruits are said to benefit people with blood type O.

4. Nuts and Seeds: Walnuts, flaxseed, and pumpkin seeds are all wonderful options. They include healthy fats and other nutrients that are appropriate for the blood type O profile.

5. Beans and Lentils: Include black-eyed peas and green lentils. They provide an excellent source of plant-based protein.

Foods to Avoid for Blood Type O Diet

1. Wheat items: Reduce or eliminate wheat-based items like bread and pasta. Individuals with blood type O may find them more difficult to digest.

2. Dairy: Limit your dairy intake, particularly milk and cheese. Consider alternatives such as almond or coconut milk.

3. Certain Grains: Avoid corn and barley. These may not be compatible with the blood type O digestive system.

4. Legumes: Some legumes are helpful, while others, such as lentils and kidney beans, may be incompatible with a blood type O diet.

5. Processed Foods: Avoid processed and highly refined foods. Choose complete, natural foods to promote general wellness.

SHOPPING LISTS FOR BLOOD TYPE O

Blood Type O Diet Shopping List

Proteins

- Lean beef

- Lamb
- Poultry (chicken, turkey)
- Salmon
- Mackerel

Vegetables

- Kale
- Spinach
- Broccoli
- Brussels sprouts
- Sweet potatoes

Fruits

- Berries (blueberries, strawberries)
- Cherries
- Plums
- Pineapple
- Papaya

Nuts and Seeds

- Walnuts
- Flaxseeds
- Pumpkin seeds
- Almonds

Beans and Lentils

- Black-eyed peas
- Green lentils

Dairy Alternatives

- Almond milk
- Coconut milk

Grains

- Quinoa
- Rice (brown or wild rice)
- Rye (in moderation)

Healthy Fats

- Olive oil
- Avocado

Herbs and Spices

- Ginger
- Turmeric
- Garlic
- Parsley
- Basil

TIPS FOR A SUCCESSFUL BLOOD TYPE O DIET

1. Prioritize Protein: Make lean protein a staple of your meals to boost your metabolism and muscular health.
2. Veggies: Focus on dark, leafy greens and cruciferous veggies for their high nutritional value.
3. Choose Beneficial Fruits: Focus on fruits that correspond to the Blood Type O guidelines, particularly berries and cherries.
4. Include Healthy Fats: For long-lasting energy, include sources of healthy fats such as olive oil and almonds.
5. Mindful Cooking Methods: To keep nutritional content, choose grilling, baking, or steaming over frying.
6. Stay Hydrated: Drink lots of water throughout the day to promote digestion and general health.
7. Read Labels: Avoid processed foods and carefully read labels to verify that items comply with the Blood Type O requirements.
8. Moderate Exercise: Exercise regularly at a moderate intensity to supplement your diet and improve your general health.

CHAPTER 2: 30-DAY MEAL PLAN

DAY 1

BREAKFAST: Omelet with Spinach and Turkey

LUNCH: Grilled Chicken and Vegetable Salad

SNACK: Turkey and Veggie Roll-Ups

DINNER: Grilled Lemon Garlic Chicken with Roasted Vegetables

DAY 2

BREAKFAST: Greek Yogurt Parfait with Berries

LUNCH: Salmon and Quinoa Bowl with Lemon-Dill Dressing

SNACK: Apple and Almond Butter Slices

DINNER: Spiced Turkey and Quinoa Stuffed Bell Peppers

DAY 3

BREAKFAST: Sweet Potato and Turkey Hash

LUNCH: Turkey and Avocado Wrap with Greens

SNACK: Spicy Edamame

DINNER: Turkey and Vegetable Stir-Fry with Ginger-Soy Sauce

DAY 4

BREAKFAST: Quinoa Breakfast Bowl

LUNCH: Eggplant and Chickpea Salad Bowl

SNACK: Cucumber and Smoked Salmon Bites

DINNER: Lemon Herb Grilled Chicken Salad

DAY 5

BREAKFAST: Egg and Spinach Breakfast Wrap

LUNCH: Lentil and Vegetable Stuffed Bell Peppers

SNACK: Almond Butter Banana Bites

DINNER: Beef and Broccoli Stir-Fry with Garlic-Ginger Sauce

DAY 6

BREAKFAST: Salmon and Avocado Toast

LUNCH: Shrimp and Zucchini Noodle Stir-Fry

SNACK: Avocado and Tomato Salsa

DINNER: Grilled Shrimp and Zucchini Skewers with Lemon-Herb Marinade

DAY 7

BREAKFAST: Banana Almond Butter Smoothie Bowl

LUNCH: Chicken and Broccoli Quinoa Bowl

SNACK: Roasted Red Pepper Hummus Stuffed Mini Bell Peppers

DINNER: Sweet Potato and Turkey Chili

DAY 8

BREAKFAST: Turkey and Sweet Potato Breakfast Hash

LUNCH: Tuna and Avocado Lettuce Wraps

SNACK: Crispy Chickpea and Rosemary Popcorn Mix

DINNER: Lemon Herb Baked Cod with Roasted Brussels Sprouts

DAY 9

BREAKFAST: Spinach and Mushroom Breakfast Quesadilla

LUNCH: Beef and Vegetable Stir-Fry with Cauliflower Rice

SNACK: Baked Zucchini Chips

DINNER: Chicken and Vegetable Stir-Fry with Cashew Nuts

DAY 10

BREAKFAST: Pumpkin Spice Chia Pudding Parfait

LUNCH: Turkey and Sweet Potato Hash

SNACK: Cajun Roasted Nuts

DINNER: Turkey and Spinach Stuffed Bell Peppers

DAY 11

BREAKFAST: Egg and Vegetable Breakfast Muffins

LUNCH: Salmon and Asparagus Foil Packets

SNACK: Mango and Chili Lime Salsa with Jicama Slices

DINNER: Sesame Ginger Chicken Stir-Fry with Vegetables

DAY 12

BREAKFAST: Apple Cinnamon Quinoa Breakfast Bowl

LUNCH: Chicken and Kale Caesar Salad

SNACK: Cucumber and Smoked Salmon Bites

DINNER: Lemon Garlic Shrimp with Quinoa and Roasted Vegetables

DAY 13

BREAKFAST: Turkey and Vegetable Breakfast Burrito

LUNCH: Egg and Turkey Spinach Wrap

SNACK: Almond Butter Banana Bites

DINNER: Lemon Herb Grilled Chicken with Asparagus

DAY 14

BREAKFAST: Blueberry Almond Breakfast Quinoa

LUNCH: Miso-Ginger Salmon Bowl

SNACK: Avocado and Tomato Salsa

DINNER: Turkey and Vegetable Skillet with Cauliflower Rice

DAY 15

BREAKFAST: Mushroom and Spinach Breakfast Frittata

LUNCH: Quinoa and Black Bean Stuffed Peppers

SNACK: Baked Zucchini Chips

DINNER: Spicy Shrimp and Broccoli Stir-Fry with Quinoa

DAY 16

BREAKFAST: Omelet with Spinach and Turkey

LUNCH: Grilled Chicken and Vegetable Salad

SNACK: Turkey and Veggie Roll-Ups

DINNER: Grilled Lemon Garlic Chicken with Roasted Vegetables

DAY 17

BREAKFAST: Greek Yogurt Parfait with Berries

LUNCH: Salmon and Quinoa Bowl with Lemon-Dill Dressing

SNACK: Apple and Almond Butter Slices

DINNER: Spiced Turkey and Quinoa Stuffed Bell Peppers

DAY 18

BREAKFAST: Sweet Potato and Turkey Hash

LUNCH: Turkey and Avocado Wrap with Greens

SNACK: Spicy Edamame

DINNER: Turkey and Vegetable Stir-Fry with Ginger-Soy Sauce

DAY 19

BREAKFAST: Quinoa Breakfast Bowl

LUNCH: Eggplant and Chickpea Salad Bowl

SNACK: Cucumber and Smoked Salmon Bites

DINNER: Lemon Herb Grilled Chicken Salad

DAY 20

BREAKFAST: Egg and Spinach Breakfast Wrap

LUNCH: Lentil and Vegetable Stuffed Bell Peppers

SNACK: Almond Butter Banana Bites

DINNER: Beef and Broccoli Stir-Fry with Garlic-Ginger Sauce

DAY 21

BREAKFAST: Salmon and Avocado Toast

LUNCH: Shrimp and Zucchini Noodle Stir-Fry

SNACK: Avocado and Tomato Salsa

DINNER: Grilled Shrimp and Zucchini Skewers with Lemon-Herb Marinade

DAY 22

BREAKFAST: Banana Almond Butter Smoothie Bowl

LUNCH: Chicken and Broccoli Quinoa Bowl

SNACK: Roasted Red Pepper Hummus Stuffed Mini Bell Peppers

DINNER: Sweet Potato and Turkey Chili

DAY 23

BREAKFAST: Turkey and Sweet Potato Breakfast Hash

LUNCH: Tuna and Avocado Lettuce Wraps

SNACK: Crispy Chickpea and Rosemary Popcorn Mix

DINNER: Lemon Herb Baked Cod with Roasted Brussels Sprouts

DAY 24

BREAKFAST: Spinach and Mushroom Breakfast Quesadilla

LUNCH: Beef and Vegetable Stir-Fry with Cauliflower Rice

SNACK: Baked Zucchini Chips

DINNER: Chicken and Vegetable Stir-Fry with Cashew Nuts

DAY 25

BREAKFAST: Pumpkin Spice Chia Pudding Parfait

LUNCH: Turkey and Sweet Potato Hash

SNACK: Cajun Roasted Nuts

DINNER: Turkey and Spinach Stuffed Bell Peppers

DAY 26

BREAKFAST: Egg and Vegetable Breakfast Muffins

LUNCH: Salmon and Asparagus Foil Packets

SNACK: Mango and Chili Lime Salsa with Jicama Slices

DINNER: Sesame Ginger Chicken Stir-Fry with Vegetables

DAY 27

BREAKFAST: Apple Cinnamon Quinoa Breakfast Bowl

LUNCH: Chicken and Kale Caesar Salad

SNACK: Cucumber and Smoked Salmon Bites

DINNER: Lemon Garlic Shrimp with Quinoa and Roasted Vegetables

DAY 28

BREAKFAST: Turkey and Vegetable Breakfast Burrito

LUNCH: Egg and Turkey Spinach Wrap

SNACK: Almond Butter Banana Bites

DINNER: Lemon Herb Grilled Chicken with Asparagus

DAY 29

BREAKFAST: Blueberry Almond Breakfast Quinoa

LUNCH: Miso-Ginger Salmon Bowl

SNACK: Avocado and Tomato Salsa

DINNER: Turkey and Vegetable Skillet with Cauliflower Rice

DAY 30

BREAKFAST: Mushroom and Spinach Breakfast Frittata

LUNCH: Quinoa and Black Bean Stuffed Peppers

SNACK: Baked Zucchini Chips

DINNER: Spicy Shrimp and Broccoli Stir-Fry with Quinoa

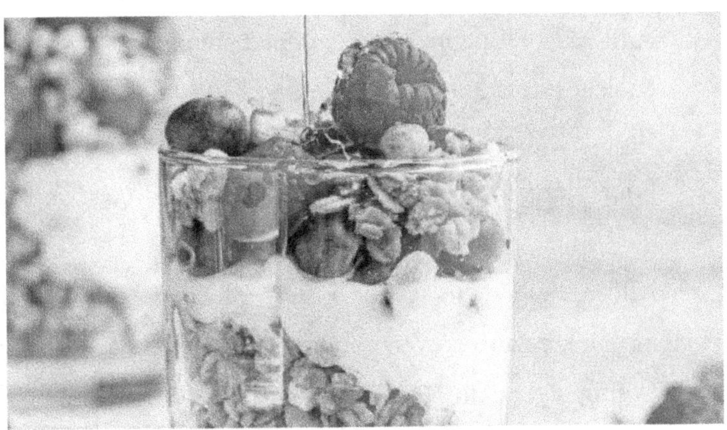

Omelet with Spinach and Turkey

Ingredients:

- 2 large eggs
- 1/4 cup diced turkey (cooked)
- 1/2 cup fresh spinach, chopped
- 1/4 cup red bell pepper, diced
- 1 tablespoon olive oil
- Salt and pepper to taste

Directions:

1. In a bowl, beat the eggs and season with a pinch of salt and pepper.
2. Heat olive oil in a non-stick skillet over medium heat.

3. Add diced turkey and sauté for 2-3 minutes until it starts to brown.

4. Add red bell pepper and chopped spinach to the skillet, cook for an additional 2 minutes until the vegetables are slightly softened.

5. Pour the beaten eggs over the turkey and vegetables in the skillet.

6. Allow the eggs to set for a moment, then gently stir the mixture, ensuring even cooking.

7. Continue cooking until the eggs are fully set and the veggies are tender.

8. Slide the omelet onto a plate and fold it in half for a delicious and nutritious breakfast.

Greek Yogurt Parfait with Berries

Ingredients:

- 1 cup plain Greek yogurt (unsweetened)
- 1/2 cup mixed berries (blueberries, strawberries, or raspberries)
- 1 tablespoon chia seeds
- 1 tablespoon chopped walnuts
- 1 teaspoon honey (optional)
- A dash of cinnamon

Directions:

1. In a bowl or glass, start with a layer of Greek yogurt.

2. Add a layer of mixed berries on top of the yogurt.

3. Sprinkle chia seeds and chopped walnuts over the berries.

4. Drizzle honey on top if desired for added sweetness.

5. Repeat the layers until you've used all the ingredients.

6. Finish with a sprinkle of cinnamon for extra flavor.

7. Serve immediately and enjoy this delicious and nutrient-packed breakfast.

Sweet Potato and Turkey Hash

Ingredients:

- 1 medium sweet potato, peeled and grated
- 1/2 cup diced turkey (cooked)
- 1/4 cup red onion, finely chopped
- 1 clove garlic, minced
- 1 tablespoon olive oil
- 1/2 teaspoon paprika
- Salt and pepper to taste
- Fresh parsley for garnish (optional)

Directions:

1. Heat olive oil in a skillet over medium heat.

2. Add minced garlic and chopped red onion, sauté until softened.

3. Add grated sweet potato to the skillet, stirring occasionally until it begins to crisp.

4. Incorporate diced turkey, paprika, salt, and pepper into the mixture.

5. Cook for an additional 5-7 minutes, allowing flavors to meld and sweet potato to cook through.

6. Once everything is cooked and well-mixed, transfer to a plate.

7. Garnish with fresh parsley if desired.

8. Serve warm and savor this flavorful, Blood Type O-friendly breakfast.

Quinoa Breakfast Bowl

Ingredients:

- 1/2 cup cooked quinoa
- 1/4 cup diced avocado
- 1/4 cup cherry tomatoes, halved
- 1/4 cup cucumber, diced
- 2 tablespoons feta cheese, crumbled
- 1 tablespoon olive oil
- Fresh lemon juice
- Salt and pepper to taste

- Chopped fresh herbs (such as basil or parsley) for garnish

Directions:

1. In a bowl, combine cooked quinoa, diced avocado, cherry tomatoes, and cucumber.
2. Drizzle olive oil over the mixture and squeeze fresh lemon juice for a zesty flavor.
3. Add salt and pepper to taste, adjusting according to your preference.
4. Toss the ingredients gently to ensure even distribution of flavors.
5. Sprinkle crumbled feta cheese on top of the quinoa mixture.
6. Garnish with chopped fresh herbs for added freshness.
7. Serve immediately and relish this nutrient-packed, Blood Type O-friendly breakfast bowl.

Egg and Spinach Breakfast Wrap

Ingredients:

- 2 large eggs
- 1 cup fresh spinach, chopped
- 1/4 cup diced bell pepper (any color)
- 2 whole-grain tortillas
- 1 tablespoon olive oil

- Salt and pepper to taste
- Salsa or hot sauce (optional)

Directions:

1. In a skillet, heat olive oil over medium heat.
2. Add diced bell pepper and sauté until slightly softened.
3. Add chopped spinach to the skillet and cook until wilted.
4. In a separate bowl, whisk the eggs and season with salt and pepper.
5. Pour the beaten eggs over the veggies in the skillet.
6. Scramble the eggs with the vegetables until fully cooked.
7. Warm the tortillas in the skillet or microwave for a few seconds.
8. Spoon the egg and vegetable mixture onto each tortilla.
9. Optionally, add salsa or hot sauce for extra flavor.
10. Roll up the tortillas into wraps and serve immediately.

Salmon and Avocado Toast

Ingredients:

- 2 slices of whole-grain bread
- 1/2 avocado, mashed
- 4 oz smoked salmon
- 1 tablespoon cream cheese (optional)
- Lemon wedges for garnish
- Fresh dill or chives for garnish

- Salt and pepper to taste

Directions:

1. Toast the slices of whole-grain bread to your liking.

2. Spread mashed avocado evenly on each slice.

3. If desired, add a thin layer of cream cheese on top of the avocado.

4. Gently layer smoked salmon over the avocado and cream cheese.

5. Sprinkle salt and pepper to taste.

6. Garnish with fresh dill or chives for added freshness.

7. Squeeze lemon wedges over the top for a citrusy kick.

8. Serve immediately and savor this delicious and Omega-3 rich breakfast.

Banana Almond Butter Smoothie Bowl

Ingredients:

- 1 ripe banana
- 2 tablespoons almond butter
- 1/2 cup unsweetened almond milk
- 1/4 cup rolled oats
- 1 tablespoon chia seeds
- Handful of sliced strawberries for topping
- 1 tablespoon chopped almonds for topping
- Drizzle of honey (optional)

Directions:

1. In a blender, combine the ripe banana, almond butter, almond milk, rolled oats, and chia seeds.
2. Blend until smooth and creamy.
3. Pour the smoothie into a bowl.
4. Top with sliced strawberries and chopped almonds.
5. If desired, drizzle honey over the top for a touch of sweetness.
6. Enjoy this nutrient-rich and Blood Type O-friendly smoothie bowl.

Turkey and Sweet Potato Breakfast Hash

Ingredients:

- 1 cup sweet potatoes, peeled and diced
- 1/2 cup diced turkey (cooked)
- 1/4 cup red onion, finely chopped
- 1 clove garlic, minced
- 1 tablespoon olive oil
- 1/2 teaspoon smoked paprika
- Salt and pepper to taste
- 2 eggs (optional, for topping)
- Fresh parsley for garnish

Directions:

1. Heat olive oil in a skillet over medium heat.

2. Add minced garlic and chopped red onion, sauté until softened.

3. Add diced sweet potatoes to the skillet and cook until they start to brown and are cooked through.

4. Incorporate diced turkey, smoked paprika, salt, and pepper into the mixture.

5. Cook for an additional 5-7 minutes, allowing flavors to meld.

6. If desired, create wells in the hash and crack an egg into each well. Cover and cook until eggs are done to your liking.

7. Garnish with fresh parsley for added freshness.

8. Serve hot, and enjoy this flavorful and hearty breakfast hash.

Spinach and Mushroom Breakfast Quesadilla

Ingredients:

- 2 whole-grain tortillas
- 1 cup fresh spinach, chopped
- 1/2 cup mushrooms, sliced
- 1/4 cup red bell pepper, diced

- 1/2 cup shredded mozzarella cheese
- 1 tablespoon olive oil
- Salt and pepper to taste
- Salsa or guacamole for dipping (optional)

Directions:

1. In a skillet, heat olive oil over medium heat.
2. Add sliced mushrooms and diced red bell pepper, sauté until mushrooms are browned.
3. Add chopped spinach to the skillet, cooking until wilted.
4. Remove the vegetables from the skillet and set aside.
5. Place one tortilla in the skillet, sprinkle half of the shredded mozzarella on top.
6. Add the sautéed vegetables over the cheese, then top with the remaining cheese.
7. Place the second tortilla on top and press down gently.
8. Cook for 2-3 minutes on each side or until the tortilla is golden brown and the cheese is melted.
9. Remove from the skillet, let it cool for a moment, then slice into wedges.
10. Serve with salsa or guacamole for dipping, if desired.

Pumpkin Spice Chia Pudding Parfait

Ingredients:

- 3 tablespoons chia seeds

- 1 cup unsweetened almond milk
- 1/4 cup canned pumpkin puree
- 1 tablespoon maple syrup (or sweetener of choice)
- 1/2 teaspoon pumpkin spice blend
- 1/4 cup granola
- 1/4 cup pomegranate seeds
- Greek yogurt (optional, for layering)
- Crushed nuts (such as pecans or almonds) for topping

Directions:

1. In a bowl, mix chia seeds, almond milk, pumpkin puree, maple syrup, and pumpkin spice.
2. Stir well and let it sit in the refrigerator for at least 2 hours or overnight until it thickens.
3. Once the chia pudding has set, start layering in a glass or bowl.
4. Begin with a layer of chia pudding, followed by a layer of granola.
5. Add a layer of pomegranate seeds, and if desired, a layer of Greek yogurt.
6. Repeat the layers until you've used all the ingredients.
7. Top with crushed nuts for added crunch.
8. Serve chilled and enjoy this festive and Blood Type O-friendly Pumpkin Spice Chia Pudding Parfait.

Egg and Vegetable Breakfast Muffins

Ingredients:

- 4 large eggs
- 1/2 cup diced bell peppers (any color)
- 1/2 cup cherry tomatoes, quartered
- 1/4 cup red onion, finely chopped
- 1/4 cup spinach, chopped
- 1/4 cup feta cheese, crumbled
- 1 tablespoon olive oil
- Salt and pepper to taste
- Fresh herbs (such as chives or parsley) for garnish

Directions:

1. Preheat the oven to 350°F (175°C). Grease a muffin tin or use paper liners.
2. In a skillet, heat olive oil over medium heat.
3. Add diced bell peppers and chopped red onion, sauté until softened.
4. Add cherry tomatoes and spinach, cooking until spinach wilts.
5. In a bowl, beat the eggs and season with salt and pepper.
6. Stir the sautéed vegetables into the beaten eggs.
7. Pour the egg and vegetable mixture evenly into the muffin cups.
8. Sprinkle crumbled feta cheese on top of each muffin.

9. Bake in the preheated oven for 15-20 minutes or until the eggs are set.

10. Garnish with fresh herbs and let them cool slightly before serving.

Apple Cinnamon Quinoa Breakfast Bowl

Ingredients:

- 1/2 cup cooked quinoa
- 1 medium apple, diced
- 2 tablespoons chopped walnuts
- 1 teaspoon cinnamon
- 1 tablespoon almond butter
- 1 tablespoon honey (optional)
- 1/4 cup unsweetened almond milk
- A sprinkle of chia seeds (optional)

Directions:

1. In a bowl, combine the cooked quinoa, diced apple, and chopped walnuts.
2. Sprinkle cinnamon over the mixture and stir well.
3. Warm the almond butter slightly and drizzle it over the quinoa mixture.
4. If desired, add honey for sweetness.
5. Pour unsweetened almond milk over the top.

6. Optionally, sprinkle chia seeds for an extra nutritional boost.

7. Stir everything together to combine the flavors.

8. Serve immediately and enjoy this flavorful Apple Cinnamon Quinoa Breakfast Bowl.

Turkey and Vegetable Breakfast Burrito

Ingredients:

- 1 whole-grain tortilla
- 1/2 cup diced turkey (cooked)
- 1/4 cup black beans, drained and rinsed
- 2 tablespoons diced red onion
- 2 tablespoons diced tomatoes
- 1/4 cup shredded cheddar cheese
- 1 tablespoon chopped cilantro
- 1/2 avocado, sliced
- Salsa for topping (optional)
- Salt and pepper to taste

Directions:

1. Warm the whole-grain tortilla in a skillet or microwave for a few seconds.

2. In the center of the tortilla, layer diced turkey, black beans, red onion, diced tomatoes, and shredded cheddar cheese.

3. Sprinkle chopped cilantro over the filling.

4. Add slices of avocado on top.

5. Season with salt and pepper to taste.

6. Fold the sides of the tortilla over the filling and roll it into a burrito.

7. If desired, warm the assembled burrito in the skillet for a couple of minutes.

8. Top with salsa if you like an extra kick.

9. Serve immediately and relish this satisfying and protein-packed Turkey and Vegetable Breakfast Burrito.

Blueberry Almond Breakfast Quinoa

Ingredients:

- 1/2 cup cooked quinoa
- 1/2 cup fresh blueberries
- 2 tablespoons almond butter
- 1 tablespoon chopped almonds
- 1 tablespoon maple syrup
- 1/4 teaspoon vanilla extract
- A pinch of cinnamon
- Unsweetened almond milk (optional, for serving)

Directions:

1. In a bowl, combine the cooked quinoa, fresh blueberries, and chopped almonds.

2. In a small saucepan, warm the almond butter, maple syrup, and vanilla extract over low heat until well combined.

3. Pour the almond butter mixture over the quinoa and berries, stirring to coat evenly.

4. Sprinkle a pinch of cinnamon for added flavor.

5. If desired, serve with a splash of unsweetened almond milk for a creamier consistency.

6. Stir everything together and adjust sweetness to taste.

7. Serve immediately and enjoy this wholesome and Blood Type O-friendly Blueberry Almond Breakfast Quinoa.

Mushroom and Spinach Breakfast Frittata

Ingredients:

- 4 large eggs
- 1 cup fresh spinach, chopped
- 1/2 cup mushrooms, sliced
- 1/4 cup red bell pepper, diced
- 1/4 cup feta cheese, crumbled
- 1 tablespoon olive oil
- Salt and pepper to taste
- Fresh herbs (such as parsley or thyme) for garnish

Directions:

1. Preheat the oven to 350°F (175°C).

2. In an oven-safe skillet, heat olive oil over medium heat.

3. Add sliced mushrooms and diced red bell pepper, sautéing until mushrooms are browned.

4. Add chopped spinach to the skillet, cooking until wilted.

5. In a bowl, beat the eggs and season with salt and pepper.

6. Pour the beaten eggs over the vegetables in the skillet.

7. Sprinkle crumbled feta cheese evenly over the eggs.

8. Cook on the stovetop for 2-3 minutes until the edges start to set.

9. Transfer the skillet to the preheated oven and bake for about 12-15 minutes or until the frittata is set in the center.

10. Garnish with fresh herbs, slice into wedges, and serve warm.

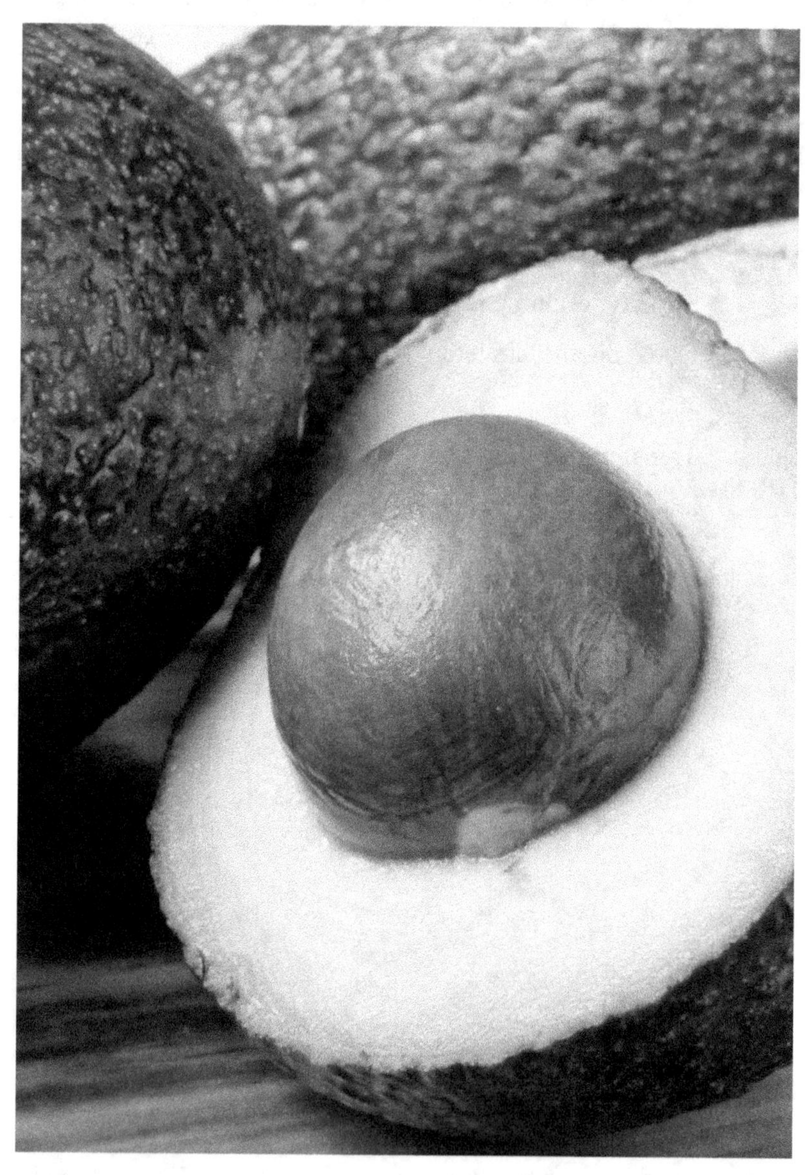

CHAPTER 4: LUNCH

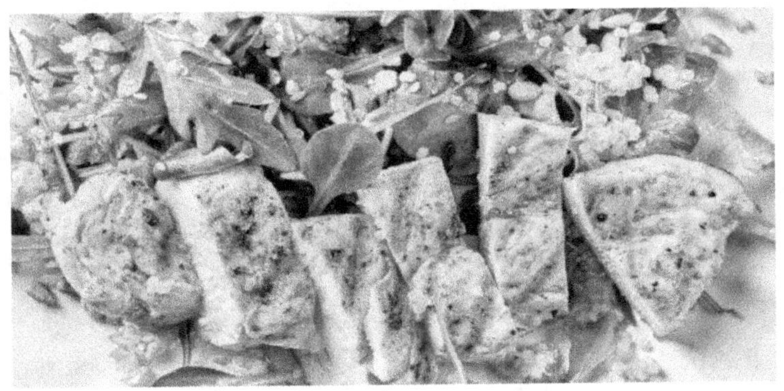

Grilled Chicken and Vegetable Salad

Ingredients:

- 1 boneless, skinless chicken breast
- 2 cups mixed salad greens (e.g., spinach, arugula, romaine)
- 1 cup cherry tomatoes, halved
- 1/2 cucumber, sliced
- 1/4 cup red onion, thinly sliced
- 1/4 cup bell peppers, diced (any color)
- 2 tablespoons olive oil
- 1 tablespoon balsamic vinegar
- 1 teaspoon Dijon mustard
- Salt and pepper to taste
- Fresh herbs (such as basil or parsley) for garnish

Directions:

1. Preheat the grill or grill pan over medium-high heat.
2. Season the chicken breast with salt and pepper.
3. Grill the chicken for about 6-8 minutes per side or until cooked through and juices run clear.
4. While the chicken is grilling, prepare the salad by combining mixed greens, cherry tomatoes, cucumber, red onion, and bell peppers in a large bowl.
5. In a small bowl, whisk together olive oil, balsamic vinegar, Dijon mustard, salt, and pepper to create the dressing.
6. Once the chicken is cooked, let it rest for a few minutes before slicing it into thin strips.
7. Add the grilled chicken strips to the salad.
8. Drizzle the dressing over the salad and toss gently to coat evenly.
9. Garnish with fresh herbs for added flavor.
10. Serve immediately and enjoy this light and nutritious Grilled Chicken and Vegetable Salad.

Salmon and Quinoa Bowl with Lemon–Dill Dressing

Ingredients:

- 1 cup cooked quinoa

- 6 oz wild-caught salmon filet
- 1 cup broccoli florets
- 1/2 cup shredded carrots
- 1/4 cup sliced red cabbage
- 1 tablespoon olive oil
- Salt and pepper to taste
- Fresh lemon wedges for garnish

Lemon-Dill Dressing:

- 2 tablespoons olive oil
- 1 tablespoon fresh lemon juice
- 1 teaspoon Dijon mustard
- 1 tablespoon fresh dill, chopped
- Salt and pepper to taste

Directions:

1. Preheat the oven to 400°F (200°C).
2. Place the salmon filet on a baking sheet lined with parchment paper.
3. Season the salmon with salt, pepper, and a drizzle of olive oil.
4. Roast the salmon in the preheated oven for about 12-15 minutes or until it flakes easily with a fork.
5. While the salmon is cooking, steam the broccoli until tender-crisp.

6. In a bowl, combine cooked quinoa, steamed broccoli, shredded carrots, and sliced red cabbage.

7. In a separate small bowl, whisk together the ingredients for the Lemon-Dill Dressing.

8. Once the salmon is done, flake it into bite-sized pieces.

9. Add the flaked salmon to the quinoa and vegetable mixture.

10. Drizzle the Lemon-Dill Dressing over the bowl and toss gently to combine.

11. Garnish with fresh lemon wedges for an extra burst of flavor.

12. Serve warm and enjoy this delicious and Omega-3 rich Salmon and Quinoa Bowl.

Turkey and Avocado Wrap with Greens

Ingredients:
- 1 whole-grain wrap or tortilla
- 1/2 cup cooked and shredded turkey
- 1/4 cup black beans, drained and rinsed
- 1/4 cup cherry tomatoes, halved
- 1/2 avocado, sliced
- 1 cup mixed salad greens (e.g., arugula, spinach)
- 1 tablespoon olive oil
- 1 tablespoon balsamic vinegar

- Salt and pepper to taste

Directions:

1. In a bowl, toss the mixed salad greens with olive oil, balsamic vinegar, salt, and pepper.
2. Warm the whole-grain wrap in a skillet or microwave for a few seconds.
3. In the center of the wrap, layer shredded turkey, black beans, cherry tomatoes, and avocado slices.
4. Spoon the dressed salad greens over the turkey and vegetable filling.
5. Fold the sides of the wrap over the filling and roll it into a wrap.
6. Optionally, warm the assembled wrap in the skillet for a couple of minutes.
7. Slice in half and serve immediately.

Eggplant and Chickpea Salad Bowl

Ingredients:

- 1 medium-sized eggplant, diced
- 1 can (15 oz) chickpeas, drained and rinsed
- 1 cup cherry tomatoes, halved
- 1/4 cup red onion, finely chopped
- 2 tablespoons olive oil
- 1 teaspoon ground cumin

- 1 teaspoon smoked paprika
- Salt and pepper to taste
- 2 cups mixed salad greens (e.g., romaine, arugula)
- 1/4 cup crumbled feta cheese
- Lemon wedges for garnish

Directions:

1. Preheat the oven to 400°F (200°C).
2. In a bowl, toss diced eggplant with olive oil, ground cumin, smoked paprika, salt, and pepper.
3. Spread the seasoned eggplant on a baking sheet and roast in the preheated oven for about 20-25 minutes or until golden and tender.
4. While the eggplant is roasting, assemble the salad by combining chickpeas, cherry tomatoes, and red onion in a large bowl.
5. Once the eggplant is done, add it to the salad mixture.
6. Toss everything together until well combined.
7. Arrange mixed salad greens in serving bowls or plates.
8. Spoon the eggplant and chickpea mixture over the greens.
9. Sprinkle crumbled feta cheese on top for added flavor.
10. Garnish with lemon wedges for a refreshing touch.
11. Serve immediately and enjoy this flavorful and protein-rich Eggplant and Chickpea Salad Bowl.

Lentil and Vegetable Stuffed Bell Peppers

Ingredients:

- 2 large bell peppers (any color)
- 1 cup cooked lentils
- 1/2 cup cherry tomatoes, diced
- 1/4 cup red onion, finely chopped
- 1/4 cup feta cheese, crumbled
- 2 tablespoons olive oil
- 1 teaspoon dried oregano
- 1/2 teaspoon ground cumin
- Salt and pepper to taste
- Fresh parsley for garnish

Directions:

1. Preheat the oven to 375°F (190°C).
2. Cut the tops off the bell peppers and remove the seeds and membranes.
3. In a bowl, combine cooked lentils, diced cherry tomatoes, red onion, feta cheese, olive oil, dried oregano, ground cumin, salt, and pepper.
4. Stuff each bell pepper with the lentil and vegetable mixture.
5. Place the stuffed peppers in a baking dish.
6. Bake in the preheated oven for about 25-30 minutes or until the peppers are tender.

7. Once done, remove from the oven and let them cool slightly.

8. Garnish with fresh parsley before serving.

Shrimp and Zucchini Noodle Stir-Fry

Ingredients:

- 8 oz shrimp, peeled and deveined
- 2 medium-sized zucchinis, spiralized into noodles
- 1 cup snap peas, ends trimmed
- 1 red bell pepper, thinly sliced
- 2 tablespoons coconut aminos (or soy sauce)
- 1 tablespoon sesame oil
- 1 tablespoon olive oil
- 1 teaspoon grated ginger
- 2 cloves garlic, minced
- Salt and pepper to taste
- Sesame seeds and chopped green onions for garnish

Directions:

1. In a wok or large skillet, heat olive oil over medium-high heat.

2. Add shrimp and stir-fry for 2-3 minutes or until they turn pink and opaque. Remove from the wok and set aside.

3. In the same wok, add sesame oil and sauté grated ginger and minced garlic until fragrant.

4. Add spiralized zucchini, snap peas, and sliced red bell pepper to the wok. Stir-fry for about 3-4 minutes until vegetables are crisp-tender.

5. Return the cooked shrimp to the wok and toss to combine with the vegetables.

6. Pour coconut aminos (or soy sauce) over the mixture and stir well to coat evenly.

7. Season with salt and pepper to taste.

8. Cook for an additional 2 minutes, ensuring everything is heated through.

9. Garnish with sesame seeds and chopped green onions before serving.

Chicken and Broccoli Quinoa Bowl

Ingredients:
- 1 cup cooked quinoa
- 6 oz boneless, skinless chicken breast, thinly sliced
- 1 cup broccoli florets
- 1/4 cup sliced carrots
- 2 tablespoons soy sauce or tamari
- 1 tablespoon olive oil
- 1 teaspoon honey
- 1 teaspoon grated ginger
- 1 clove garlic, minced

- Sesame seeds and sliced green onions for garnish

Directions:

1. In a wok or skillet, heat olive oil over medium-high heat.
2. Add thinly sliced chicken to the wok and stir-fry until browned and cooked through.
3. Add broccoli florets and sliced carrots to the wok, continuing to stir-fry for another 3-4 minutes until veggies are tender-crisp.
4. In a small bowl, whisk together soy sauce (or tamari), honey, grated ginger, and minced garlic.
5. Pour the sauce over the chicken and vegetables in the wok. Stir to coat evenly.
6. Cook for an additional 2 minutes, ensuring everything is well combined and heated through.
7. In serving bowls, layer the cooked quinoa as the base.
8. Spoon the chicken and vegetable stir-fry over the quinoa.
9. Garnish with sesame seeds and sliced green onions.
10. Serve immediately and enjoy this flavorful and protein-packed Chicken and Broccoli Quinoa Bowl.

Tuna and Avocado Lettuce Wraps

Ingredients:

- 1 can (5 oz) tuna, drained
- 1/2 avocado, mashed

- 1/4 cup diced cucumber

- 1/4 cup cherry tomatoes, halved

- 2 tablespoons red onion, finely chopped

- 1 tablespoon olive oil

- 1 tablespoon lemon juice

- Salt and pepper to taste

- Large lettuce leaves for wrapping (e.g., iceberg or romaine)

Directions:

1. In a bowl, combine drained tuna, mashed avocado, diced cucumber, cherry tomatoes, and chopped red onion.

2. In a separate small bowl, whisk together olive oil, lemon juice, salt, and pepper to create the dressing.

3. Pour the dressing over the tuna and vegetable mixture and toss gently to combine.

4. Wash and pat dry large lettuce leaves, using them as wraps.

5. Spoon the tuna and avocado mixture onto each lettuce leaf.

6. Fold the sides of the lettuce leaf over the filling and roll it into a wrap.

7. Arrange the wraps on a plate and serve immediately.

Beef and Vegetable Stir-Fry with Cauliflower Rice

Ingredients:

- 8 oz lean beef strips
- 1 cup broccoli florets
- 1/2 red bell pepper, thinly sliced
- 1/2 yellow bell pepper, thinly sliced
- 1/2 cup snow peas, ends trimmed
- 1 cup cauliflower rice
- 2 tablespoons coconut aminos (or soy sauce)
- 1 tablespoon olive oil
- 1 teaspoon grated ginger
- 2 cloves garlic, minced
- Salt and pepper to taste
- Sesame seeds for garnish

Directions:

1. In a large skillet or wok, heat olive oil over medium-high heat.
2. Add lean beef strips and stir-fry until browned and cooked to your liking.
3. Remove the cooked beef from the skillet and set it aside.
4. In the same skillet, add grated ginger and minced garlic, sautéing until fragrant.

5. Add broccoli, red bell pepper, yellow bell pepper, and snow peas to the skillet. Stir-fry for about 3-4 minutes until vegetables are crisp-tender.

6. Push the vegetables to the side and add cauliflower rice to the skillet.

7. Cook cauliflower rice for 2-3 minutes, stirring occasionally.

8. Combine the cooked beef back into the skillet with the vegetables and cauliflower rice.

9. Pour coconut aminos (or soy sauce) over the mixture, tossing everything to combine.

10. Season with salt and pepper to taste.

11. Cook for an additional 2 minutes to ensure everything is heated through.

12. Garnish with sesame seeds before serving.

Turkey and Sweet Potato Hash

Ingredients:

- 1 lb ground turkey
- 2 medium sweet potatoes, peeled and diced
- 1/2 red onion, finely chopped
- 1 bell pepper, diced (any color)
- 2 cloves garlic, minced
- 1 teaspoon smoked paprika

- 1/2 teaspoon ground cumin
- Salt and pepper to taste
- 2 tablespoons olive oil
- Fresh cilantro for garnish

Directions:

1. In a large skillet, heat olive oil over medium-high heat.
2. Add ground turkey and cook until browned, breaking it apart with a spoon.
3. Once the turkey is browned, add diced sweet potatoes to the skillet.
4. Cook for about 10-12 minutes or until the sweet potatoes are tender and slightly crispy.
5. Add chopped red onion, bell pepper, minced garlic, smoked paprika, ground cumin, salt, and pepper to the skillet.
6. Stir to combine all the ingredients and cook for an additional 5-7 minutes until the vegetables are softened.
7. Adjust seasoning to taste.
8. Garnish with fresh cilantro before serving.

Salmon and Asparagus Foil Packets

Ingredients:

- 2 salmon filets
- 1 bunch asparagus, trimmed

- 1 lemon, sliced
- 2 tablespoons olive oil
- 2 cloves garlic, minced
- 1 teaspoon dried dill
- Salt and pepper to taste
- Fresh parsley for garnish

Directions:

1. Preheat the oven to 400°F (200°C).
2. Tear two large pieces of aluminum foil and place them on a baking sheet.
3. In the center of each foil piece, place a salmon filet and a handful of trimmed asparagus.
4. Drizzle olive oil over each salmon filet and asparagus bundle.
5. Sprinkle minced garlic and dried dill evenly over the salmon and asparagus.
6. Season with salt and pepper to taste.
7. Place lemon slices on top of each salmon filet.
8. Fold the foil over the salmon and asparagus, creating sealed packets.
9. Bake in the preheated oven for about 15-20 minutes or until the salmon is cooked through and flakes easily.
10. Carefully open the foil packets, garnish with fresh parsley, and serve.

Chicken and Kale Caesar Salad

Ingredients:

- 8 oz grilled chicken breast, sliced
- 4 cups kale, stems removed and chopped
- 1 cup cherry tomatoes, halved
- 1/4 cup Parmesan cheese, shaved
- 1/4 cup pumpkin seeds (pepitas)
- 1/2 cup Caesar dressing (look for a Blood Type O-friendly option or make your own)
- Salt and pepper to taste
- Lemon wedges for garnish

Directions:

1. In a large bowl, combine chopped kale, sliced grilled chicken, cherry tomatoes, Parmesan cheese, and pumpkin seeds.
2. Drizzle Caesar dressing over the salad.
3. Toss the salad until the ingredients are well coated with the dressing.
4. Season with salt and pepper to taste.
5. Divide the salad onto serving plates.
6. Garnish with additional shaved Parmesan and a wedge of lemon on each plate.
7. Serve immediately and enjoy this flavorful and nutrient-packed Chicken and Kale Caesar Salad.

Egg and Turkey Spinach Wrap

Ingredients:

- 2 large eggs
- 1/2 cup ground turkey, cooked
- 1 cup fresh spinach leaves
- 1/4 cup red bell pepper, diced
- 1 tablespoon olive oil
- Salt and pepper to taste
- 1 whole-grain wrap or tortilla

Directions:

1. In a skillet, heat olive oil over medium heat.
2. Add diced red bell pepper and sauté until softened.
3. Add ground turkey to the skillet and cook until browned.
4. Push the turkey and pepper mixture to one side of the skillet.
5. Crack the eggs into the empty side of the skillet and scramble until fully cooked.
6. Combine the scrambled eggs with the turkey and pepper mixture.
7. Add fresh spinach to the skillet and toss until wilted.
8. Season with salt and pepper to taste.
9. Warm the whole-grain wrap in the skillet or microwave for a few seconds.

10. Spoon the egg, turkey, and spinach mixture onto the center of the wrap.

11. Fold the sides of the wrap over the filling and roll it into a wrap.

12. Slice in half and serve immediately.

Miso-Ginger Salmon Bowl

Ingredients:

- 2 salmon filets
- 1 cup cooked brown rice
- 1 cup broccoli florets
- 1/2 cup shredded carrots
- 2 tablespoons miso paste
- 1 tablespoon low-sodium soy sauce
- 1 tablespoon rice vinegar
- 1 tablespoon grated ginger
- 1 tablespoon sesame oil
- Sesame seeds and green onions for garnish

Directions:

1. Preheat the oven to 400°F (200°C).

2. Place salmon filets on a baking sheet lined with parchment paper.

3. In a small bowl, mix miso paste, soy sauce, rice vinegar, grated ginger, and sesame oil to create the marinade.

4. Brush the salmon filets with the miso-ginger marinade, ensuring they are well coated.

5. Bake in the preheated oven for about 15-20 minutes or until the salmon is cooked through and flakes easily.

6. While the salmon is baking, steam the broccoli until tender-crisp.

7. In serving bowls, assemble the cooked brown rice, steamed broccoli, and shredded carrots.

8. Once the salmon is done, place it on top of the rice and vegetables.

9. Garnish with sesame seeds and sliced green onions.

10. Serve warm and enjoy this flavorful and nutrient-rich Miso-Ginger Salmon Bowl.

Quinoa and Black Bean Stuffed Peppers

Ingredients:
- 4 large bell peppers (any color)
- 1 cup cooked quinoa
- 1 can (15 oz) black beans, drained and rinsed
- 1 cup corn kernels (fresh or frozen)
- 1 cup diced tomatoes
- 1/2 cup red onion, finely chopped
- 1 teaspoon ground cumin
- 1 teaspoon chili powder

- Salt and pepper to taste
- 1 cup shredded cheddar cheese
- Fresh cilantro for garnish

Directions:

1. Preheat the oven to 375°F (190°C).
2. Cut the tops off the bell peppers and remove the seeds and membranes.
3. In a large bowl, combine cooked quinoa, black beans, corn, diced tomatoes, red onion, ground cumin, chili powder, salt, and pepper.
4. Spoon the quinoa and black bean mixture into each bell pepper until they are filled.
5. Place the stuffed peppers in a baking dish.
6. Top each stuffed pepper with shredded cheddar cheese.
7. Bake in the preheated oven for about 25-30 minutes or until the peppers are tender and the cheese is melted and bubbly.
8. Once done, remove from the oven and let them cool slightly.
9. Garnish with fresh cilantro before serving.

CHAPTER 5: SNACKS AND DESSERTS

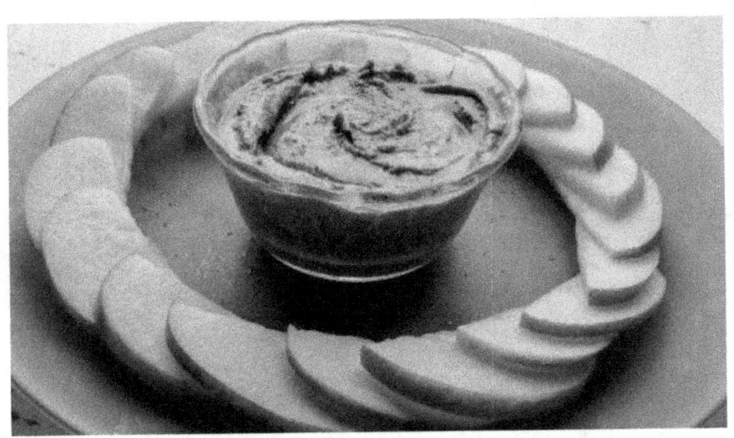

Turkey and Veggie Roll-Ups

Ingredients:

- 4 slices nitrate-free turkey breast
- 1/2 cup hummus (choose a Blood Type O-friendly variety or make your own)
- 1 medium cucumber, julienned
- 1 medium carrot, julienned
- 1/2 avocado, sliced
- Fresh basil leaves (optional)
- Salt and pepper to taste

Directions:

1. Lay out the turkey slices on a clean surface.

2. Spread a thin layer of hummus evenly over each turkey slice.

3. Place julienned cucumber and carrot strips along one edge of each turkey slice.

4. Add a slice of avocado and, if desired, fresh basil leaves on top of the veggies.

5. Sprinkle with a pinch of salt and pepper for added flavor.

6. Carefully roll up each turkey slice, starting from the edge with the veggies.

7. Secure each roll-up with a toothpick if needed.

8. Slice the rolled-up turkey into bite-sized pieces.

9. Arrange the Turkey and Veggie Roll-Ups on a plate and serve.

Apple and Almond Butter Slices

Ingredients:

- 1 medium apple, cored and sliced
- 2 tablespoons almond butter (check for Blood Type O-friendly options or make your own)
- 1 tablespoon chia seeds
- 1 tablespoon chopped walnuts
- Cinnamon for sprinkling

Directions:

1. Core and slice the apple into thin rounds.

2. Spread a thin layer of almond butter on each apple slice.

3. Sprinkle chia seeds and chopped walnuts evenly over the almond butter.

4. Lightly dust the slices with cinnamon for added flavor.

5. Arrange the Apple and Almond Butter Slices on a plate.

6. Serve immediately and enjoy this crunchy and nutritious snack.

Spicy Edamame

Ingredients:

- 1 cup frozen edamame, thawed
- 1 tablespoon olive oil
- 1 teaspoon chili powder
- 1/2 teaspoon smoked paprika
- 1/4 teaspoon garlic powder
- Salt to taste
- Lime wedges for serving

Directions:

1. Preheat the oven to 375°F (190°C).

2. In a bowl, toss thawed edamame with olive oil, chili powder, smoked paprika, garlic powder, and salt.

3. Spread the seasoned edamame on a baking sheet lined with parchment paper.

4. Bake in the preheated oven for about 15-20 minutes or until the edamame are slightly crispy, stirring halfway through.

5. Remove from the oven and let them cool for a few minutes.

6. Transfer the Spicy Edamame to a serving bowl.

7. Squeeze lime wedges over the edamame for a zesty kick.

8. Serve immediately and enjoy this flavorful and protein-packed snack.

Cucumber and Smoked Salmon Bites

Ingredients:

- 1 large cucumber, sliced into rounds
- 4 oz smoked salmon, cut into small pieces
- 1/4 cup cream cheese (choose a Blood Type O-friendly option)
- 1 tablespoon fresh dill, chopped
- Black pepper to taste
- Lemon wedges for serving

Directions:

1. Lay out the cucumber rounds on a serving platter.

2. In a small bowl, mix cream cheese and chopped fresh dill until well combined.

3. Spread a small amount of the cream cheese mixture on each cucumber round.

4. Top each cucumber round with a piece of smoked salmon.

5. Sprinkle black pepper over the smoked salmon for added flavor.

6. Arrange the Cucumber and Smoked Salmon Bites on the serving platter.

7. Serve with lemon wedges on the side for a zesty touch.

8. Enjoy this elegant and protein-rich snack.

Almond Butter Banana Bites

Ingredients:

- 2 medium-sized bananas, peeled and sliced
- 4 tablespoons almond butter (choose a Blood Type O-friendly option or make your own)
- 2 tablespoons unsweetened shredded coconut
- 2 tablespoons chopped almonds
- Cinnamon for sprinkling

Directions:

1. Lay out the banana slices on a plate or serving dish.

2. Spoon a small amount of almond butter onto each banana slice.

3. Sprinkle unsweetened shredded coconut and chopped almonds over the almond butter.

4. Dust the bites with a pinch of cinnamon for added flavor.

5. Repeat the process for each banana slice.

6. Serve immediately and enjoy these Almond Butter Banana Bites.

Avocado and Tomato Salsa

Ingredients:

- 1 ripe avocado, diced
- 1 cup cherry tomatoes, quartered
- 1/4 cup red onion, finely chopped
- 1/4 cup fresh cilantro, chopped
- 1 tablespoon lime juice
- 1 tablespoon olive oil
- Salt and pepper to taste
- Whole-grain rice cakes or Blood Type O-friendly crackers for serving

Directions:

1. In a bowl, combine diced avocado, quartered cherry tomatoes, chopped red onion, and fresh cilantro.

2. In a small bowl, whisk together lime juice, olive oil, salt, and pepper to create the dressing.

3. Pour the dressing over the avocado and tomato mixture and gently toss to combine.

4. Adjust seasoning to taste.

5. Allow the Avocado and Tomato Salsa to sit for a few minutes to let the flavors meld.

6. Serve the salsa with whole-grain rice cakes or Blood Type O-friendly crackers.

Roasted Red Pepper Hummus Stuffed Mini Bell Peppers

Ingredients:

- 8 mini bell peppers, halved and seeds removed
- 1 cup roasted red pepper hummus (choose a Blood Type O-friendly option or make your own)
- 2 tablespoons pine nuts, toasted
- Fresh parsley for garnish

Directions:

1. Preheat the oven to 375°F (190°C).

2. Place mini bell pepper halves on a baking sheet.

3. Spoon roasted red pepper hummus into each pepper half.

4. Sprinkle toasted pine nuts over the hummus.

5. Bake in the preheated oven for about 10-12 minutes or until the peppers are slightly softened.

6. Remove from the oven and let them cool for a few minutes.

7. Garnish with fresh parsley before serving.

Crispy Chickpea and Rosemary Popcorn Mix

Ingredients:

- 1 cup canned chickpeas, drained and rinsed
- 2 tablespoons olive oil
- 1 teaspoon dried rosemary
- 1/2 teaspoon garlic powder
- Salt and pepper to taste
- 4 cups air-popped popcorn

Directions:

1. Preheat the oven to 400°F (200°C).

2. Pat the chickpeas dry with a paper towel and place them on a baking sheet.

3. Drizzle olive oil over the chickpeas and sprinkle with dried rosemary, garlic powder, salt, and pepper.

4. Toss the chickpeas to coat them evenly with the seasoning.

5. Roast in the preheated oven for about 20-25 minutes or until the chickpeas are crispy, shaking the pan occasionally for even cooking.

6. While the chickpeas are roasting, prepare the air-popped popcorn.

7. Once the chickpeas are done, let them cool for a few minutes.

8. In a large bowl, mix the crispy chickpeas with the air-popped popcorn.

9. Adjust salt and pepper to taste.

10. Serve this Crispy Chickpea and Rosemary Popcorn Mix as a satisfying and crunchy snack.

Baked Zucchini Chips

Ingredients:

- 2 medium-sized zucchinis, thinly sliced
- 2 tablespoons olive oil
- 1 teaspoon dried oregano
- 1/2 teaspoon garlic powder
- Salt and pepper to taste
- 2 tablespoons grated Parmesan cheese (optional)

Directions:

1. Preheat the oven to 375°F (190°C).

2. In a large bowl, toss thinly sliced zucchinis with olive oil, dried oregano, garlic powder, salt, and pepper.

3. Arrange the zucchini slices on a baking sheet in a single layer.

4. Bake in the preheated oven for about 15-20 minutes or until the zucchini chips are golden and crispy, flipping them halfway through.

5. If using Parmesan cheese, sprinkle it over the zucchini chips during the last 5 minutes of baking.

6. Remove from the oven and let the chips cool for a few minutes.

7. Serve these Baked Zucchini Chips as a delightful and healthy snack.

Cajun Roasted Nuts

Ingredients:

- 1 cup mixed nuts (almonds, walnuts, pecans)
- 1 tablespoon olive oil
- 1 teaspoon Cajun seasoning
- 1/2 teaspoon smoked paprika
- 1/4 teaspoon cayenne pepper (adjust to taste)
- Salt to taste

Directions:

1. Preheat the oven to 350°F (175°C).

2. In a bowl, toss the mixed nuts with olive oil, Cajun seasoning, smoked paprika, cayenne pepper, and salt.

3. Spread the seasoned nuts on a baking sheet in a single layer.

4. Roast in the preheated oven for about 10-15 minutes or until the nuts are golden and fragrant, stirring occasionally for even roasting.

5. Remove from the oven and let the Cajun Roasted Nuts cool completely.

6. Once cooled, store in an airtight container.

Mango and Chili Lime Salsa with Jicama Slices

Ingredients:

- 1 ripe mango, diced
- 1/2 red onion, finely chopped
- 1 jalapeño, seeded and minced
- Juice of 2 limes
- Zest of 1 lime
- 1/4 cup fresh cilantro, chopped
- Salt to taste
- Jicama, peeled and sliced, for serving

Directions:

1. In a bowl, combine diced mango, chopped red onion, minced jalapeño, lime juice, lime zest, and chopped cilantro.

2. Mix the ingredients together until well combined.

3. Add salt to taste and adjust the level of spiciness by adding more jalapeño if desired.

4. Allow the Mango and Chili Lime Salsa to sit for a few minutes to let the flavors meld.

5. Serve the salsa with jicama slices for a refreshing and crunchy snack.

Dark Chocolate-Dipped Strawberries with Almonds

Ingredients:

- 1 cup dark chocolate chips (choose at least 70% cocoa)
- 1 tablespoon coconut oil
- 1/2 cup almonds, finely chopped
- 1 pint fresh strawberries, washed and dried

Directions:

1. Line a baking sheet with parchment paper.

2. In a microwave-safe bowl, melt the dark chocolate chips and coconut oil in 20-second intervals, stirring each time until smooth.

3. Place the finely chopped almonds in a shallow dish.

4. Holding each strawberry by the green stem, dip it into the melted chocolate, ensuring it's coated halfway.

5. Immediately dip the chocolate-covered part into the chopped almonds, rolling it to coat evenly.

6. Place the dipped strawberries on the prepared baking sheet.

7. Repeat the process for each strawberry.

8. Once all strawberries are dipped and coated, refrigerate the baking sheet for about 15-20 minutes to allow the chocolate to set.

9. Serve these Dark Chocolate-Dipped Strawberries with Almonds as a delightful and guilt-free dessert.

Coconut Chia Pudding with Fresh Berries

Ingredients:

- 1/4 cup chia seeds
- 1 cup coconut milk (unsweetened, Blood Type O-friendly)
- 1 tablespoon maple syrup or honey (optional)
- 1/2 teaspoon vanilla extract
- Fresh berries (strawberries, blueberries, raspberries) for topping
- Unsweetened shredded coconut for garnish

Directions:

1. In a bowl, combine chia seeds, coconut milk, maple syrup or honey (if using), and vanilla extract.

2. Stir the mixture well and let it sit for 5 minutes.

3. Stir the mixture again to prevent clumping of chia seeds, then cover and refrigerate for at least 2 hours or overnight.
4. Before serving, give the chia pudding a good stir to achieve a smooth consistency.
5. Spoon the Coconut Chia Pudding into serving glasses or bowls.
6. Top with fresh berries and a sprinkle of unsweetened shredded coconut.
7. Serve chilled and enjoy this creamy and nutritious dessert.

Frozen Banana and Almond Butter Bites

Ingredients:

- 2 large bananas, peeled and sliced into rounds
- 1/4 cup almond butter (choose a Blood Type O-friendly option)
- 1/4 cup unsweetened shredded coconut
- 1/4 cup chopped almonds
- Dark chocolate chips for drizzling (optional)

Directions:

1. Lay out the banana rounds on a parchment paper-lined tray.

2. Spoon a small amount of almond butter onto each banana round.

3. Sprinkle shredded coconut and chopped almonds over the almond butter.

4. Optional: Melt dark chocolate chips and drizzle over the banana rounds for added sweetness.

5. Place the tray in the freezer and let the Frozen Banana and Almond Butter Bites set for at least 2 hours.

6. Once frozen, transfer the bites to a container for storage.

7. Serve these delicious frozen bites as a cool and satisfying dessert.

Pomegranate and Mint Sorbet

Ingredients:

- 2 cups pomegranate juice (unsweetened)
- 1/4 cup fresh mint leaves, chopped
- 1 tablespoon agave nectar or honey (optional)
- Pomegranate arils for garnish

Directions:

1. In a blender, combine pomegranate juice, chopped mint leaves, and agave nectar or honey (if using).

2. Blend until the mint is finely incorporated into the juice.

3. Pour the mixture into an ice cream maker.

4. Churn according to the manufacturer's instructions until you achieve a sorbet consistency.

5. If you don't have an ice cream maker, pour the mixture into a shallow dish and place it in the freezer.

6. Every 30 minutes, stir the sorbet with a fork to break up ice crystals until it reaches the desired consistency.

7. Once the sorbet is ready, scoop into bowls or glasses.

8. Garnish with fresh pomegranate arils.

9. Serve immediately and enjoy this refreshing Pomegranate and Mint Sorbet.

Baked Cinnamon Apple Slices

Ingredients:

- 2 large apples, cored and thinly sliced
- 1 tablespoon melted coconut oil
- 1 teaspoon ground cinnamon
- 1/2 teaspoon nutmeg
- 1 tablespoon maple syrup or honey (optional)
- Chopped walnuts for garnish

Directions:

1. Preheat the oven to 375°F (190°C).

2. In a bowl, toss apple slices with melted coconut oil, ground cinnamon, nutmeg, and maple syrup or honey (if using).

3. Arrange the coated apple slices on a baking sheet in a single layer.

4. Bake in the preheated oven for about 15-20 minutes or until the apples are tender and slightly caramelized, stirring halfway through.

5. Remove from the oven and let the Baked Cinnamon Apple Slices cool for a few minutes.

6. Transfer the slices to a serving dish, and sprinkle chopped walnuts over the top.

7. Serve warm and enjoy this naturally sweet and spiced dessert.

Mint Chocolate Avocado Mousse

Ingredients:

- 2 ripe avocados
- 1/4 cup unsweetened cocoa powder
- 1/4 cup almond milk (Blood Type O-friendly)
- 1/4 cup maple syrup or honey (adjust to taste)
- 1/2 teaspoon peppermint extract
- Fresh mint leaves for garnish

Directions:

1. Scoop the flesh of the ripe avocados into a blender or food processor.

2.   Add cocoa powder, almond milk, maple syrup or honey, and peppermint extract.

3.   Blend until smooth and creamy, scraping down the sides as needed.

4.   Taste and adjust the sweetness if necessary by adding more maple syrup or honey.

5.   Once the mixture is smooth, spoon the Mint Chocolate Avocado Mousse into serving glasses or bowls.

6.   Chill in the refrigerator for at least 1-2 hours to enhance the flavors.

7.   Before serving, garnish with fresh mint leaves.

8.   Enjoy this rich and indulgent dessert guilt-free.

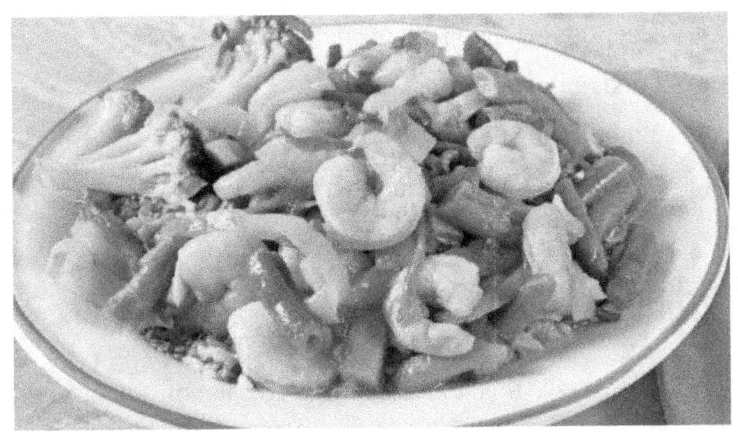

Grilled Lemon Garlic Chicken with Roasted Vegetables

Ingredients:

For the Chicken:

- 4 boneless, skinless chicken breasts
- 2 tablespoons olive oil
- Juice of 1 lemon
- 3 cloves garlic, minced
- 1 teaspoon dried oregano
- Salt and black pepper to taste

For the Roasted Vegetables:

- 2 cups broccoli florets

- 2 cups cherry tomatoes, halved
- 1 red bell pepper, sliced
- 1 yellow bell pepper, sliced
- 1 red onion, sliced
- 2 tablespoons olive oil
- 1 teaspoon dried thyme
- Salt and black pepper to taste

Directions:

1. Preheat the grill to medium-high heat.

2. In a bowl, mix together olive oil, lemon juice, minced garlic, dried oregano, salt, and black pepper to create the marinade for the chicken.

3. Place the chicken breasts in a resealable plastic bag or shallow dish and coat them with the marinade. Let it marinate in the refrigerator for at least 30 minutes.

4. While the chicken is marinating, preheat the oven to 400°F (200°C).

5. In a large bowl, combine broccoli florets, halved cherry tomatoes, sliced red and yellow bell peppers, sliced red onion, olive oil, dried thyme, salt, and black pepper. Toss to coat the vegetables evenly.

6. Spread the vegetables on a baking sheet in a single layer. Roast in the preheated oven for about 20-25 minutes or until they are tender and slightly caramelized.

7. Grill the marinated chicken breasts on the preheated grill for approximately 6-8 minutes per side or until fully cooked and no longer pink in the center.

8. Serve the Grilled Lemon Garlic Chicken over a bed of the roasted vegetables.

9. Garnish with fresh herbs like parsley or basil if desired.

10. Enjoy this delicious and nutritious Grilled Lemon Garlic Chicken with Roasted Vegetables.

Spiced Turkey and Quinoa Stuffed Bell Peppers

Ingredients:

For the Stuffed Bell Peppers:

- 4 large bell peppers, halved and seeds removed
- 1 cup quinoa, rinsed
- 2 cups water or vegetable broth
- 1 pound ground turkey
- 1 onion, finely chopped
- 2 cloves garlic, minced
- 1 teaspoon ground cumin
- 1 teaspoon smoked paprika
- 1/2 teaspoon chili powder
- Salt and black pepper to taste
- 1 can (15 oz) black beans, drained and rinsed

- 1 cup corn kernels (fresh or frozen)
- 1 cup diced tomatoes

For Garnish:

- Fresh cilantro, chopped
- Avocado slices
- Lime wedges

Directions:

1. Preheat the oven to 375°F (190°C).

2. In a medium saucepan, combine quinoa and water or vegetable broth. Bring to a boil, then reduce heat, cover, and simmer for 15-20 minutes or until quinoa is cooked and liquid is absorbed.

3. While the quinoa is cooking, heat olive oil in a large skillet over medium heat. Add chopped onion and garlic, sauté until softened.

4. Add ground turkey to the skillet and cook until browned. Drain any excess fat.

5. Season the turkey mixture with ground cumin, smoked paprika, chili powder, salt, and black pepper. Stir to combine.

6. In a large mixing bowl, combine the cooked quinoa, seasoned turkey mixture, black beans, corn, and diced tomatoes.

7. Stuff each bell pepper half with the turkey and quinoa mixture.

8. Place the stuffed bell peppers in a baking dish and cover with foil.

9. Bake in the preheated oven for 25-30 minutes or until the peppers are tender.

10. Garnish with fresh cilantro and serve with avocado slices and lime wedges.

11. Enjoy these Spiced Turkey and Quinoa Stuffed Bell Peppers as a flavorful and wholesome dinner option.

Turkey and Vegetable Stir-Fry with Ginger-Soy Sauce

Ingredients:

- 1 pound ground turkey
- 2 tablespoons olive oil
- 1 onion, thinly sliced
- 2 bell peppers (any color), thinly sliced
- 2 cups broccoli florets
- 3 carrots, julienned
- 3 cloves garlic, minced
- 1 tablespoon fresh ginger, grated
- 1/4 cup low-sodium soy sauce (or Tamari for a gluten-free option)

- 1 tablespoon rice vinegar
- 1 tablespoon honey
- 1 teaspoon sesame oil
- Sesame seeds for garnish (optional)
- Green onions, sliced, for garnish

Directions:

1. In a large skillet or wok, heat olive oil over medium-high heat.
2. Add ground turkey to the skillet and cook until browned. Drain any excess fat.
3. Push the turkey to one side of the skillet, add a bit more oil if needed, and sauté onions, bell peppers, broccoli, and carrots until they start to soften.
4. Stir in minced garlic and grated ginger, cooking for an additional minute until fragrant.
5. In a small bowl, whisk together soy sauce, rice vinegar, honey, and sesame oil.
6. Pour the sauce over the turkey and vegetables in the skillet. Toss everything together until well-coated and heated through.
7. Garnish with sesame seeds and sliced green onions.
8. Serve this Turkey and Vegetable Stir-Fry over steamed brown rice or cauliflower rice and enjoy!

Lemon Herb Grilled Chicken Salad

Ingredients:

For the Grilled Chicken:

- 4 boneless, skinless chicken breasts
- 2 tablespoons olive oil
- Zest and juice of 1 lemon
- 2 cloves garlic, minced
- 1 teaspoon dried thyme
- Salt and black pepper to taste

For the Salad:

- Mixed salad greens (lettuce, spinach, arugula)
- Cherry tomatoes, halved
- Cucumber, sliced
- Red onion, thinly sliced
- Avocado, sliced
- Feta cheese, crumbled (optional)

For the Lemon Herb Dressing:

- 1/4 cup olive oil
- Zest and juice of 1 lemon
- 1 tablespoon Dijon mustard
- 1 teaspoon honey
- 1 teaspoon dried oregano
- Salt and black pepper to taste

Directions:

1. Preheat the grill to medium-high heat.

2. In a bowl, mix together olive oil, lemon zest, lemon juice, minced garlic, dried thyme, salt, and black pepper for the marinade.

3. Place the chicken breasts in a resealable plastic bag or shallow dish and coat them with the marinade. Let it marinate in the refrigerator for at least 30 minutes.

4. Grill the marinated chicken breasts on the preheated grill for approximately 6-8 minutes per side or until fully cooked and no longer pink in the center.

5. While the chicken is grilling, prepare the salad by arranging mixed greens, cherry tomatoes, cucumber, red onion, and avocado on a serving platter.

6. In a small bowl, whisk together olive oil, lemon zest, lemon juice, Dijon mustard, honey, dried oregano, salt, and black pepper for the dressing.

7. Once the chicken is done, slice it into strips.

8. Arrange the grilled chicken strips over the prepared salad.

9. Drizzle the Lemon Herb Dressing over the salad and chicken.

10. Optionally, sprinkle crumbled feta cheese over the top.

11. Serve and enjoy this refreshing Lemon Herb Grilled Chicken Salad.

Beef and Broccoli Stir-Fry with Garlic-Ginger Sauce

Ingredients:

- 1 pound flank steak, thinly sliced
- 2 tablespoons olive oil
- 4 cups broccoli florets
- 1 red bell pepper, thinly sliced
- 4 cloves garlic, minced
- 1 tablespoon fresh ginger, grated
- 1/4 cup low-sodium soy sauce (or Tamari for a gluten-free option)
- 1 tablespoon oyster sauce
- 1 tablespoon rice vinegar
- 1 tablespoon honey
- 1 teaspoon sesame oil
- 2 tablespoons water
- Sesame seeds for garnish (optional)
- Green onions, sliced, for garnish

Directions:

1. In a large skillet or wok, heat olive oil over medium-high heat.

2. Add thinly sliced flank steak to the skillet and cook until browned. Remove the cooked steak from the skillet and set aside.

3. In the same skillet, add a bit more oil if needed, and sauté broccoli florets and red bell pepper until they start to soften.

4. Stir in minced garlic and grated ginger, cooking for an additional minute until fragrant.

5. In a small bowl, whisk together soy sauce, oyster sauce, rice vinegar, honey, sesame oil, and water.

6. Add the cooked steak back to the skillet and pour the sauce over the beef and vegetables. Toss everything together until well-coated and heated through.

7. Garnish with sesame seeds and sliced green onions.

8. Serve and enjoy this Beef and Broccoli Stir-Fry over steamed brown rice or cauliflower rice.

Grilled Shrimp and Zucchini Skewers with Lemon-Herb Marinade

Ingredients:

- 1 pound large shrimp, peeled and deveined
- 2 zucchini, sliced into rounds
- 2 tablespoons olive oil
- Zest and juice of 1 lemon

- 2 cloves garlic, minced

- 1 teaspoon dried thyme

- 1 teaspoon dried rosemary

- Salt and black pepper to taste

- Wooden skewers, soaked in water for 30 minutes

Directions:

1. Preheat the grill to medium-high heat.

2. In a bowl, mix together olive oil, lemon zest, lemon juice, minced garlic, dried thyme, dried rosemary, salt, and black pepper to create the marinade.

3. Thread the marinated shrimp and zucchini slices onto the soaked wooden skewers, alternating between shrimp and zucchini.

4. Place the skewers on the preheated grill and cook for 2-3 minutes per side or until the shrimp are opaque and the zucchini is tender.

5. Baste the skewers with the remaining marinade during grilling.

6. Once cooked, remove the skewers from the grill and let them rest for a few minutes.

7. Serve these Grilled Shrimp and Zucchini Skewers with a side of mixed greens or your favorite salad.

8. Garnish with additional lemon slices and fresh herbs if desired.

Sweet Potato and Turkey Chili

Ingredients:

- 1 pound ground turkey
- 2 sweet potatoes, peeled and diced
- 1 onion, diced
- 2 cloves garlic, minced
- 1 can (15 oz) kidney beans, drained and rinsed
- 1 can (15 oz) diced tomatoes
- 1 can (6 oz) tomato paste
- 3 cups low-sodium chicken or vegetable broth
- 2 teaspoons chili powder
- 1 teaspoon cumin
- 1 teaspoon smoked paprika
- Salt and black pepper to taste
- Olive oil for cooking
- Optional toppings: shredded cheddar cheese, Greek yogurt, sliced green onions

Directions:

1. In a large pot, heat olive oil over medium-high heat.
2. Add diced sweet potatoes and sauté for 5 minutes until slightly softened.
3. Add diced onions and minced garlic, continue sautéing for another 3-5 minutes until the onions are translucent.

4. Add ground turkey to the pot, breaking it apart with a spoon, and cook until browned.

5. Stir in chili powder, cumin, smoked paprika, salt, and black pepper.

6. Pour in diced tomatoes, kidney beans, tomato paste, and chicken or vegetable broth. Stir well to combine.

7. Bring the chili to a boil, then reduce the heat to low, cover, and let it simmer for 20-25 minutes until sweet potatoes are tender.

8. Taste and adjust the seasoning if needed.

9. Serve this delicious Sweet Potato and Turkey Chili hot, topped with shredded cheddar cheese, a dollop of Greek yogurt, and sliced green onions if desired.

Lemon Herb Baked Cod with Roasted Brussels Sprouts

Ingredients:

For the Baked Cod:

- 4 cod filets
- 2 tablespoons olive oil
- Zest and juice of 1 lemon
- 2 cloves garlic, minced
- 1 teaspoon dried thyme
- 1 teaspoon dried rosemary

- Salt and black pepper to taste

For the Roasted Brussels Sprouts:

- 1 pound Brussels sprouts, trimmed and halved

- 2 tablespoons olive oil

- Salt and black pepper to taste

Directions:

1. Preheat the oven to 400°F (200°C).

2. In a bowl, mix together olive oil, lemon zest, lemon juice, minced garlic, dried thyme, dried rosemary, salt, and black pepper to create the marinade for the cod.

3. Place the cod filets in a baking dish and coat them with the marinade. Let it marinate for about 15 minutes.

4. While the cod is marinating, toss halved Brussels sprouts with olive oil, salt, and black pepper. Spread them on a baking sheet.

5. Place the marinated cod filets in the same oven for 15-20 minutes or until the fish is cooked through and easily flakes with a fork.

6. Roast the Brussels sprouts in the preheated oven for approximately 20-25 minutes or until they are golden and crispy on the edges.

7. Serve the Lemon Herb Baked Cod over a bed of roasted Brussels sprouts.

8. Garnish with additional lemon slices and fresh herbs if desired.

Chicken and Vegetable Stir-Fry with Cashew Nuts

Ingredients:

- 1 pound boneless, skinless chicken breasts, thinly sliced
- 2 tablespoons olive oil
- 1 onion, thinly sliced
- 1 red bell pepper, thinly sliced
- 1 yellow bell pepper, thinly sliced
- 2 cups broccoli florets
- 1 cup snap peas, trimmed
- 3 cloves garlic, minced
- 1 tablespoon fresh ginger, grated
- 1/4 cup low-sodium soy sauce (or Tamari for a gluten-free option)
- 2 tablespoons oyster sauce
- 1 tablespoon rice vinegar
- 1 tablespoon honey
- 1 teaspoon sesame oil
- 1 cup unsalted cashew nuts
- Green onions, sliced, for garnish

Directions:

1. In a large skillet or wok, heat olive oil over medium-high heat.

2. Add thinly sliced chicken to the skillet and cook until browned and cooked through. Remove the cooked chicken from the skillet and set aside.

3. In the same skillet, add a bit more oil if needed, and sauté sliced onion, red bell pepper, yellow bell pepper, broccoli, and snap peas until they start to soften.

4. Stir in minced garlic and grated ginger, cooking for an additional minute until fragrant.

5. In a small bowl, whisk together soy sauce, oyster sauce, rice vinegar, honey, and sesame oil.

6. Add the cooked chicken back to the skillet, pour the sauce over the chicken and vegetables. Toss everything together until well-coated and heated through.

7. In a separate pan, lightly toast the cashew nuts over medium heat for 2-3 minutes until fragrant and golden.

8. Stir in the toasted cashew nuts into the stir-fry.

9. Garnish with sliced green onions.

10. Serve this Chicken and Vegetable Stir-Fry over steamed brown rice or cauliflower rice and enjoy!

Turkey and Spinach Stuffed Bell Peppers

Ingredients:

- 4 large bell peppers, halved and seeds removed
- 1 pound ground turkey
- 1 onion, finely chopped
- 2 cloves garlic, minced
- 2 cups fresh spinach, chopped
- 1 can (15 oz) diced tomatoes, drained
- 1 cup cooked quinoa
- 1 teaspoon dried oregano
- 1 teaspoon dried basil
- Salt and black pepper to taste
- 1 cup shredded mozzarella cheese

Directions:

1. Preheat the oven to 375°F (190°C).
2. In a large skillet, cook ground turkey over medium heat until browned. Drain any excess fat.
3. Add chopped onions and minced garlic to the skillet, sauté until onions are softened.
4. Stir in chopped spinach and cook until wilted.
5. Add drained diced tomatoes, cooked quinoa, dried oregano, dried basil, salt, and black pepper. Mix well.
6. Fill each bell pepper half with the turkey and spinach mixture.

7. Place the stuffed bell peppers in a baking dish.

8. Sprinkle shredded mozzarella cheese on top of each stuffed pepper.

9. Cover the baking dish with foil and bake in the preheated oven for 25-30 minutes or until the peppers are tender.

10. Remove the foil and broil for an additional 2-3 minutes to melt and brown the cheese.

11. Serve these Turkey and Spinach Stuffed Bell Peppers and enjoy!

Sesame Ginger Chicken Stir-Fry with Vegetables

Ingredients:

- 1 pound boneless, skinless chicken thighs, thinly sliced
- 2 tablespoons sesame oil
- 1 onion, thinly sliced
- 1 bell pepper (any color), thinly sliced
- 2 carrots, julienned
- 2 cups snow peas, ends trimmed
- 3 cloves garlic, minced
- 1 tablespoon fresh ginger, grated
- 1/4 cup low-sodium soy sauce (or Tamari for a gluten-free option)

- 1 tablespoon oyster sauce

- 1 tablespoon rice vinegar

- 1 tablespoon honey

- 1 teaspoon sesame seeds for garnish

- Green onions, sliced, for garnish

- Cooked brown rice or cauliflower rice for serving

Directions:

1. In a wok or large skillet, heat sesame oil over medium-high heat.

2. Add thinly sliced chicken to the wok and cook until browned and cooked through. Remove the cooked chicken from the wok and set aside.

3. In the same wok, add a bit more oil if needed, and sauté sliced onion, bell pepper, julienned carrots, and snow peas until they start to soften.

4. Stir in minced garlic and grated ginger, cooking for an additional minute until fragrant.

5. In a small bowl, whisk together soy sauce, oyster sauce, rice vinegar, and honey.

6. Add the cooked chicken back to the wok, pour the sauce over the chicken and vegetables. Toss everything together until well-coated and heated through.

7. Optional: Toast sesame seeds in a dry pan over medium heat for 2-3 minutes until golden.

8. Serve this Sesame Ginger Chicken Stir-Fry over cooked brown rice or cauliflower rice.

9. Garnish with sesame seeds and sliced green onions.

Lemon Garlic Shrimp with Quinoa and Roasted Vegetables

Ingredients:

For the Lemon Garlic Shrimp:

- 1 pound large shrimp, peeled and deveined
- 3 tablespoons olive oil
- Zest and juice of 1 lemon
- 4 cloves garlic, minced
- 1 teaspoon dried thyme
- Salt and black pepper to taste

For the Quinoa and Roasted Vegetables:

- 1 cup quinoa, rinsed
- 2 cups mixed vegetables (e.g., cherry tomatoes, bell peppers, zucchini), chopped
- 2 tablespoons olive oil
- Salt and black pepper to taste

Directions:

1. Preheat the oven to 400°F (200°C).

2. In a bowl, mix together olive oil, lemon zest, lemon juice, minced garlic, dried thyme, salt, and black pepper for the marinade.

3. Toss the peeled and deveined shrimp in the marinade and let it sit for about 10 minutes.

4. Spread the marinated shrimp on a baking sheet lined with parchment paper.

5. In a separate bowl, mix the chopped mixed vegetables with olive oil, salt, and black pepper. Spread them on another baking sheet.

6. Roast both the shrimp and vegetables in the preheated oven for about 15-20 minutes or until the shrimp are opaque and the vegetables are tender.

7. While the shrimp and vegetables are roasting, cook quinoa according to package instructions.

8. Once cooked, fluff the quinoa with a fork.

9. Serve the Lemon Garlic Shrimp over a bed of cooked quinoa and roasted vegetables.

10. Garnish with additional lemon slices and fresh herbs if desired.

Balsamic Glazed Chicken with Roasted Brussels Sprouts and Butternut Squash

Ingredients:

For the Balsamic Glazed Chicken:

- 1.5 pounds boneless, skinless chicken breasts
- 3 tablespoons balsamic vinegar
- 2 tablespoons olive oil
- 2 tablespoons Dijon mustard
- 2 cloves garlic, minced
- 1 teaspoon dried rosemary
- Salt and black pepper to taste

For the Roasted Brussels Sprouts and Butternut Squash:

- 1 pound Brussels sprouts, trimmed and halved
- 1 small butternut squash, peeled, seeded, and cubed
- 3 tablespoons olive oil
- 1 teaspoon dried thyme
- Salt and black pepper to taste

Directions:

1. Preheat the oven to 400°F (200°C).
2. In a small bowl, whisk together balsamic vinegar, olive oil, Dijon mustard, minced garlic, dried rosemary, salt, and black pepper.

3. Place the chicken breasts in a zip-top bag or shallow dish, pour half of the balsamic mixture over them, and let it marinate for at least 15 minutes.

4. In the meantime, toss halved Brussels sprouts and cubed butternut squash with olive oil, dried thyme, salt, and black pepper on a baking sheet.

5. Place the marinated chicken breasts on the same baking sheet.

6. Roast in the preheated oven for about 25-30 minutes or until the chicken is cooked through and the vegetables are tender.

7. During the last 10 minutes of roasting, brush the remaining balsamic mixture over the chicken.

8. Once cooked, let the chicken rest for a few minutes before slicing.

9. Serve the Balsamic Glazed Chicken slices over a bed of roasted Brussels sprouts and butternut squash.

Miso-Glazed Salmon with Stir-Fried Bok Choy and Shiitake Mushrooms

Ingredients:

For the Miso-Glazed Salmon:

- 4 salmon filets
- 3 tablespoons white miso paste

- 2 tablespoons mirin (Japanese sweet rice wine)
- 1 tablespoon soy sauce
- 1 tablespoon honey
- 1 teaspoon grated fresh ginger
- Sesame seeds for garnish

For the Stir-Fried Bok Choy and Shiitake Mushrooms:

- 4 baby bok choy, sliced
- 1 cup shiitake mushrooms, sliced
- 2 tablespoons sesame oil
- 2 cloves garlic, minced
- 1 tablespoon soy sauce
- 1 teaspoon rice vinegar

Directions:

1. Preheat the oven to 400°F (200°C).
2. In a bowl, whisk together white miso paste, mirin, soy sauce, honey, and grated fresh ginger to create the miso glaze.
3. Place the salmon filets on a baking sheet lined with parchment paper.
4. Brush the miso glaze generously over the salmon fillets.
5. Roast in the preheated oven for about 12-15 minutes or until the salmon is cooked through.
6. While the salmon is roasting, heat sesame oil in a large skillet over medium-high heat.

7. Add minced garlic and stir-fry for about 30 seconds until fragrant.

8. Add sliced bok choy and shiitake mushrooms to the skillet. Stir-fry for 3-5 minutes until the vegetables are tender-crisp.

9. Drizzle soy sauce and rice vinegar over the stir-fried vegetables, toss to combine.

10. Once the salmon is cooked, serve it over a bed of stir-fried bok choy and shiitake mushrooms.

11. Garnish with sesame seeds.

12. Enjoy this delicious Miso-Glazed Salmon with Stir-Fried Bok Choy and Shiitake Mushrooms!

Lemon Herb Grilled Chicken with Asparagus

Ingredients:

- 4 boneless, skinless chicken breasts
- 3 tablespoons olive oil
- Zest and juice of 1 lemon
- 2 cloves garlic, minced
- 1 teaspoon dried oregano
- 1 teaspoon dried thyme
- Salt and black pepper to taste

For the Grilled Asparagus:

- 1 bunch asparagus, trimmed

- 2 tablespoons olive oil
- Salt and black pepper to taste

Directions:

1. Preheat the grill to medium-high heat.
2. In a bowl, whisk together olive oil, lemon zest, lemon juice, minced garlic, dried oregano, dried thyme, salt, and black pepper to create the marinade.
3. Place the chicken breasts in a zip-top bag or shallow dish, pour half of the marinade over them, and let it marinate for at least 15 minutes.
4. In the meantime, toss trimmed asparagus with olive oil, salt, and black pepper.
5. Grill the marinated chicken breasts for about 6-8 minutes per side or until fully cooked. Ensure the internal temperature reaches 165°F (74°C).
6. During the last few minutes of grilling, place the asparagus on the grill and cook until tender-crisp, turning occasionally.
7. Remove the grilled chicken and asparagus from the grill.
8. Serve the Lemon Herb Grilled Chicken over a bed of grilled asparagus.
9. Drizzle the remaining marinade over the chicken and asparagus.

Turkey and Vegetable Skillet with Cauliflower Rice

Ingredients:

- 1 pound ground turkey
- 2 tablespoons olive oil
- 1 onion, diced
- 2 bell peppers (any color), diced
- 2 zucchinis, diced
- 3 cloves garlic, minced
- 1 teaspoon smoked paprika
- 1 teaspoon ground cumin
- Salt and black pepper to taste
- 1 can (15 oz) diced tomatoes, drained
- 1 head cauliflower, grated (for cauliflower rice)
- Fresh cilantro, chopped, for garnish

Directions:

1. In a large skillet, heat olive oil over medium-high heat.
2. Add diced onion, bell peppers, and zucchinis to the skillet. Sauté until vegetables are softened.
3. Add minced garlic, smoked paprika, ground cumin, salt, and black pepper. Stir well to combine.
4. Push the vegetables to one side of the skillet and add ground turkey to the empty side. Cook until browned, breaking it apart with a spoon.

5. Once the turkey is cooked, combine it with the sautéed vegetables.

6. Stir in drained diced tomatoes and let the mixture simmer for 5-7 minutes.

7. While the mixture is simmering, grate the cauliflower to make cauliflower rice.

8. Push the turkey and vegetable mixture to the side of the skillet and add the grated cauliflower. Sauté for 5-7 minutes until the cauliflower is tender.

9. Mix the cauliflower rice with the turkey and vegetable mixture until well combined.

10. Adjust seasoning if needed and sprinkle fresh cilantro on top.

11. Serve and enjoy this Turkey and Vegetable Skillet with Cauliflower Rice!

Spicy Shrimp and Broccoli Stir-Fry with Quinoa

Ingredients:

- 1 pound large shrimp, peeled and deveined
- 2 tablespoons olive oil
- 3 cups broccoli florets
- 1 red bell pepper, thinly sliced
- 3 cloves garlic, minced

- 1 tablespoon fresh ginger, grated
- 1/4 cup low-sodium soy sauce (or Tamari for a gluten-free option)
- 2 tablespoons Sriracha sauce (adjust to taste)
- 1 tablespoon honey
- 1 tablespoon rice vinegar
- 2 cups cooked quinoa

Directions:

1. In a large wok or skillet, heat olive oil over medium-high heat.
2. Add shrimp to the wok and cook until pink and opaque. Remove the cooked shrimp and set aside.
3. In the same wok, add a bit more oil if needed, and stir-fry broccoli florets and red bell pepper until they start to soften.
4. Add minced garlic and grated ginger, cook for an additional minute until fragrant.
5. In a small bowl, whisk together soy sauce, Sriracha sauce, honey, and rice vinegar.
6. Add the cooked shrimp back to the wok, pour the sauce over the shrimp and vegetables. Toss everything together until well-coated and heated through.
7. Serve the Spicy Shrimp and Broccoli Stir-Fry over a bed of cooked quinoa.

8. Adjust Sriracha sauce to taste if you prefer more heat.

Salmon and Avocado Salad with Citrus Vinaigrette

Ingredients:

For the Salmon:

- 4 salmon filets
- 2 tablespoons olive oil
- 1 teaspoon paprika
- Salt and black pepper to taste

For the Salad:

- Mixed salad greens (arugula, spinach, or your choice)
- 2 avocados, sliced
- 1 cup cherry tomatoes, halved
- 1 cucumber, sliced
- 1/4 cup red onion, thinly sliced
- 1/4 cup feta cheese, crumbled

For the Citrus Vinaigrette:

- 1/4 cup olive oil
- Juice of 1 lemon
- Juice of 1 orange
- 1 tablespoon Dijon mustard
- 1 tablespoon honey
- Salt and black pepper to taste

Directions:

1. Preheat the oven to 400°F (200°C).

2. Place salmon filets on a baking sheet lined with parchment paper.

3. Drizzle olive oil over the salmon filets, sprinkle paprika, salt, and black pepper.

4. Bake in the preheated oven for about 12-15 minutes or until the salmon is cooked through.

5. In a large salad bowl, combine mixed salad greens, sliced avocados, cherry tomatoes, cucumber, red onion, and crumbled feta cheese.

6. In a small bowl, whisk together olive oil, lemon juice, orange juice, Dijon mustard, honey, salt, and black pepper to create the citrus vinaigrette.

7. Once the salmon is cooked, let it cool for a few minutes, then flake it into bite-sized pieces.

8. Add the flaked salmon to the salad.

9. Drizzle the citrus vinaigrette over the salad and gently toss to combine.

10. Serve the Salmon and Avocado Salad immediately for a refreshing and nutritious Blood Type O Diet-friendly dinner!

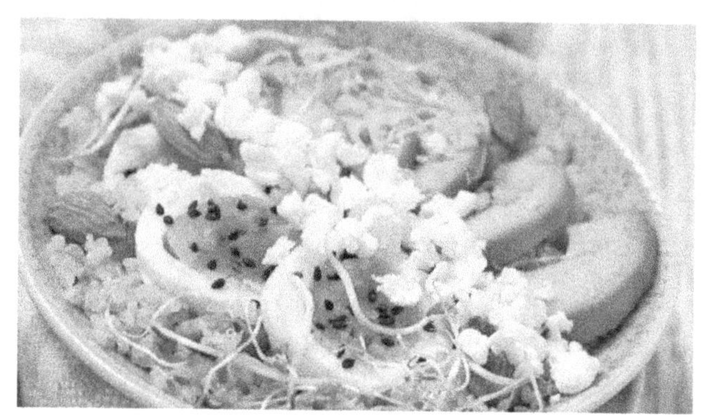

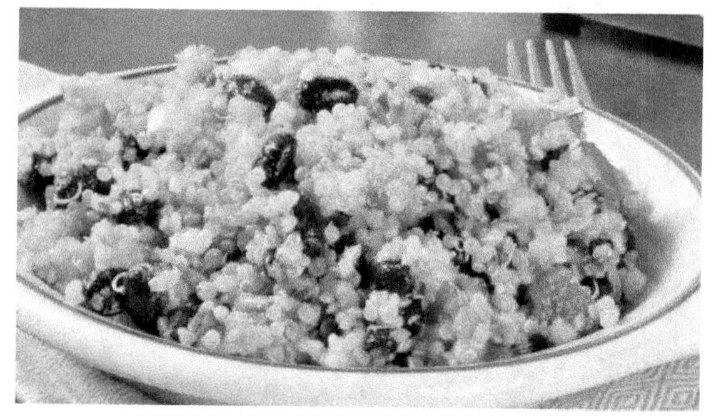

CHAPTER 7: NOURISHING SOUPS AND STEWS

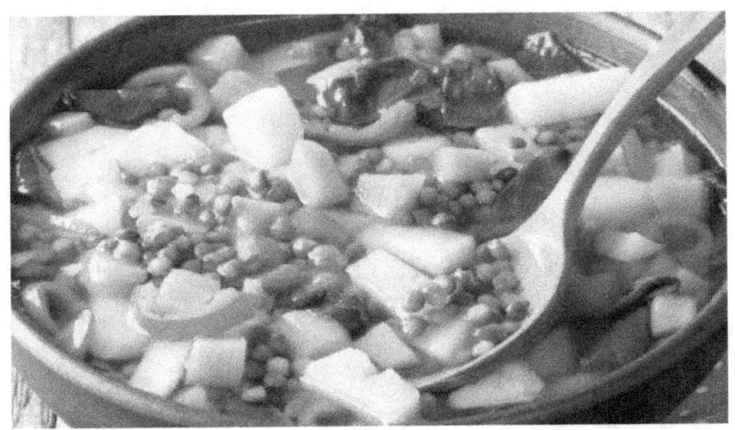

Chicken and Vegetable Soup with Turmeric

Ingredients:

- 1 pound boneless, skinless chicken breasts, diced
- 1 tablespoon olive oil
- 1 onion, diced
- 2 carrots, sliced
- 2 celery stalks, sliced
- 3 cloves garlic, minced
- 1 teaspoon ground turmeric
- 1 teaspoon dried thyme
- 6 cups chicken broth (low-sodium)

- 1 cup broccoli florets
- 1 cup kale, chopped
- Salt and black pepper to taste
- Fresh parsley, chopped, for garnish

Directions:

1. In a large pot, heat olive oil over medium-high heat.
2. Add diced chicken to the pot and cook until browned. Remove the chicken from the pot and set aside.
3. In the same pot, add diced onion, sliced carrots, and sliced celery. Sauté until the vegetables begin to soften.
4. Add minced garlic, ground turmeric, and dried thyme to the pot. Stir well to combine.
5. Pour in the chicken broth, scraping the bottom of the pot to release any flavorful bits.
6. Bring the soup to a simmer, then add back the cooked chicken.
7. Stir in broccoli florets and chopped kale. Simmer for an additional 10-15 minutes until the vegetables are tender.
8. Season the soup with salt and black pepper to taste.
9. Ladle the Chicken and Vegetable Soup into bowls.
10. Garnish with fresh chopped parsley before serving.

Spicy Lentil and Spinach Soup

Ingredients:

- 1 cup dried green or brown lentils, rinsed
- 1 tablespoon olive oil
- 1 onion, diced
- 2 carrots, sliced
- 2 celery stalks, sliced
- 3 cloves garlic, minced
- 1 teaspoon ground cumin
- 1/2 teaspoon smoked paprika
- 1/4 teaspoon cayenne pepper (adjust to taste)
- 6 cups vegetable broth (low-sodium)
- 1 can (14 oz) diced tomatoes, undrained
- 4 cups fresh spinach, chopped
- Salt and black pepper to taste
- Fresh cilantro, chopped, for garnish

Directions:

1. In a large pot, heat olive oil over medium-high heat.
2. Add diced onion, sliced carrots, and sliced celery to the pot. Sauté until the vegetables begin to soften.
3. Stir in minced garlic, ground cumin, smoked paprika, and cayenne pepper. Cook for an additional minute until fragrant.

4. Add rinsed lentils, vegetable broth, and diced tomatoes with their juice to the pot. Bring to a simmer.

5. Reduce the heat to low, cover, and let the soup simmer for about 20-25 minutes or until the lentils are tender.

6. Stir in chopped fresh spinach and let it wilt in the hot soup.

7. Season the soup with salt and black pepper to taste.

8. Ladle the Spicy Lentil and Spinach Soup into bowls.

9. Garnish with fresh chopped cilantro before serving.

Beef and Sweet Potato Stew

Ingredients:

- 1.5 pounds stewing beef, cubed
- 2 tablespoons olive oil
- 1 onion, diced
- 3 cloves garlic, minced
- 2 sweet potatoes, peeled and diced
- 3 carrots, sliced
- 2 parsnips, sliced
- 4 cups beef broth (low-sodium)
- 1 can (14 oz) diced tomatoes, undrained
- 1 teaspoon dried rosemary
- 1 teaspoon dried thyme
- Salt and black pepper to taste

- Fresh parsley, chopped, for garnish

Directions:

1. In a large pot, heat olive oil over medium-high heat.
2. Add cubed stewing beef to the pot and brown on all sides. Remove the beef from the pot and set aside.
3. In the same pot, add diced onion and minced garlic. Sauté until the onion is translucent.
4. Stir in sweet potatoes, carrots, and parsnips.
5. Return the browned beef to the pot.
6. Pour in beef broth and diced tomatoes with their juice. Add dried rosemary and dried thyme.
7. Bring the stew to a boil, then reduce the heat to low, cover, and let it simmer for about 1.5 to 2 hours or until the beef is tender.
8. Season the stew with salt and black pepper to taste.
9. Ladle the Beef and Sweet Potato Stew into bowls.
10. Garnish with fresh chopped parsley before serving.

Mushroom and Kale Miso Soup

Ingredients:

- 1 tablespoon olive oil
- 1 onion, thinly sliced
- 3 cloves garlic, minced

- 8 ounces mushrooms (shiitake, cremini, or your choice), sliced
- 4 cups vegetable broth (low-sodium)
- 2 tablespoons white miso paste
- 1 carrot, julienned
- 2 cups kale, stems removed and chopped
- 1 tablespoon soy sauce (or Tamari for a gluten-free option)
- 1 teaspoon sesame oil
- 4 green onions, sliced (for garnish)
- Sesame seeds (for garnish)

Directions:

1. In a large pot, heat olive oil over medium-high heat.
2. Add thinly sliced onion and minced garlic to the pot. Sauté until the onion is softened.
3. Add sliced mushrooms and cook until they release their moisture and become golden brown.
4. Pour in vegetable broth and bring the soup to a simmer.
5. In a small bowl, dilute miso paste with a few tablespoons of hot broth from the pot. Stir until the miso paste is well combined.
6. Add the diluted miso paste to the soup, stirring to incorporate.

7. Add julienned carrot, chopped kale, soy sauce, and sesame oil to the pot. Simmer for an additional 10-15 minutes until the vegetables are tender.

8. Adjust soy sauce to taste.

9. Ladle the Mushroom and Kale Miso Soup into bowls.

10. Garnish with sliced green onions and sprinkle sesame seeds on top.

Cabbage and Sausage Soup

Ingredients:

- 1 tablespoon olive oil
- 1 onion, diced
- 2 cloves garlic, minced
- 1 pound Italian sausage, casings removed
- 1 small head cabbage, thinly sliced
- 2 carrots, sliced
- 4 cups chicken broth (low-sodium)
- 1 can (14 oz) diced tomatoes, undrained
- 1 teaspoon dried thyme
- 1 teaspoon smoked paprika
- Salt and black pepper to taste
- Fresh parsley, chopped, for garnish

Directions:

1. In a large pot, heat olive oil over medium-high heat.

2. Add diced onion and minced garlic to the pot. Sauté until the onion is softened.

3. Add Italian sausage to the pot, breaking it apart with a spoon. Cook until browned.

4. Stir in thinly sliced cabbage and sliced carrots. Sauté for a few minutes until the vegetables start to soften.

5. Pour in chicken broth and diced tomatoes with their juice.

6. Add dried thyme and smoked paprika to the pot. Season with salt and black pepper to taste.

7. Bring the soup to a simmer and let it cook for about 15-20 minutes until the cabbage and carrots are tender.

8. Adjust seasoning if needed.

9. Ladle the Cabbage and Sausage Soup into bowls.

10. Garnish with fresh chopped parsley before serving.

Chickpea and Vegetable Stew with Turmeric

Ingredients:

- 1 tablespoon olive oil
- 1 onion, diced
- 3 cloves garlic, minced
- 2 carrots, sliced
- 2 celery stalks, sliced
- 1 bell pepper (any color), diced

- 1 teaspoon ground turmeric
- 1 teaspoon ground cumin
- 1 can (15 oz) chickpeas, drained and rinsed
- 1 can (14 oz) diced tomatoes, undrained
- 4 cups vegetable broth (low-sodium)
- 1 teaspoon dried thyme
- Salt and black pepper to taste
- Fresh cilantro, chopped, for garnish

Directions:

1. In a large pot, heat olive oil over medium-high heat.
2. Add diced onion and minced garlic to the pot. Sauté until the onion is softened.
3. Stir in sliced carrots, sliced celery, and diced bell pepper. Sauté for a few minutes until the vegetables start to soften.
4. Add ground turmeric and ground cumin to the pot. Stir well to combine.
5. Pour in chickpeas, diced tomatoes with their juice, and vegetable broth.
6. Add dried thyme, salt, and black pepper to taste.
7. Bring the stew to a simmer and let it cook for about 20-25 minutes until the vegetables are tender.
8. Adjust seasoning if needed.
9. Ladle the Chickpea and Vegetable Stew into bowls.

10. Garnish with fresh chopped cilantro before serving.

Lentil and Turkey Sausage Soup

Ingredients:

- 1 tablespoon olive oil
- 1 onion, diced
- 2 carrots, sliced
- 2 celery stalks, sliced
- 3 cloves garlic, minced
- 1 pound turkey sausage, sliced
- 1 cup dried green or brown lentils, rinsed
- 6 cups chicken broth (low-sodium)
- 1 can (14 oz) diced tomatoes, undrained
- 1 teaspoon dried oregano
- 1 teaspoon smoked paprika
- Salt and black pepper to taste
- Fresh parsley, chopped, for garnish

Directions:

1. In a large pot, heat olive oil over medium-high heat.
2. Add diced onion, sliced carrots, and sliced celery to the pot. Sauté until the vegetables begin to soften.
3. Stir in minced garlic and sliced turkey sausage. Cook until the sausage is browned.

4. Add rinsed lentils, chicken broth, diced tomatoes with their juice, dried oregano, and smoked paprika to the pot.

5. Bring the soup to a simmer and let it cook for about 25-30 minutes or until the lentils are tender.

6. Season the soup with salt and black pepper to taste.

7. Ladle the Lentil and Turkey Sausage Soup into bowls.

8. Garnish with fresh chopped parsley before serving.

Quinoa and Vegetable Stew

Ingredients:

- 1 cup quinoa, rinsed
- 2 tablespoons olive oil
- 1 onion, diced
- 2 carrots, sliced
- 2 zucchini, diced
- 3 cloves garlic, minced
- 1 can (15 oz) chickpeas, drained and rinsed
- 4 cups vegetable broth (low-sodium)
- 1 can (14 oz) diced tomatoes, undrained
- 1 teaspoon ground cumin
- 1 teaspoon dried thyme
- Salt and black pepper to taste
- Fresh parsley, chopped, for garnish

Directions:

1. In a medium pot, bring 2 cups of water to a boil. Add rinsed quinoa, reduce heat to low, cover, and simmer for 15-20 minutes or until quinoa is cooked and water is absorbed.
2. In a large pot, heat olive oil over medium-high heat.
3. Add diced onion, sliced carrots, and diced zucchini to the pot. Sauté until the vegetables begin to soften.
4. Stir in minced garlic and chickpeas. Cook for an additional minute.
5. Pour in vegetable broth, diced tomatoes with their juice, ground cumin, and dried thyme.
6. Bring the stew to a simmer and let it cook for about 15-20 minutes until the vegetables are tender.
7. Season the stew with salt and black pepper to taste.
8. Fluff the cooked quinoa with a fork and add it to the pot. Stir to combine.
9. Ladle the Quinoa and Vegetable Stew into bowls.
10. Garnish with fresh chopped parsley before serving.

Shrimp and Vegetable Coconut Soup

Ingredients:

- 1 tablespoon coconut oil
- 1 onion, thinly sliced

- 2 carrots, julienned
- 1 red bell pepper, thinly sliced
- 3 cloves garlic, minced
- 1 teaspoon grated ginger
- 1 pound shrimp, peeled and deveined
- 1 can (14 oz) coconut milk
- 4 cups vegetable broth (low-sodium)
- 1 tablespoon fish sauce
- 1 tablespoon lime juice
- 1 teaspoon red curry paste
- 1 zucchini, spiralized or thinly sliced
- Salt and black pepper to taste
- Fresh cilantro, chopped, for garnish

Directions:

1. In a large pot, melt coconut oil over medium-high heat.

2. Add thinly sliced onion, julienned carrots, and sliced red bell pepper to the pot. Sauté until the vegetables begin to soften.

3. Stir in minced garlic and grated ginger. Cook for an additional minute until fragrant.

4. Add peeled and deveined shrimp to the pot. Cook until they turn pink.

5. Pour in coconut milk, vegetable broth, fish sauce, lime juice, and red curry paste. Bring the soup to a simmer.

6. Add spiralized or thinly sliced zucchini to the pot. Simmer for an additional 5-7 minutes until the zucchini is tender.

7. Season the soup with salt and black pepper to taste.

8. Ladle the Shrimp and Vegetable Coconut Soup into bowls.

9. Garnish with fresh chopped cilantro before serving.

Turkey and Butternut Squash Stew

Ingredients:

- 1.5 pounds ground turkey
- 2 tablespoons olive oil
- 1 onion, diced
- 3 cloves garlic, minced
- 1 butternut squash, peeled and diced
- 2 carrots, sliced
- 4 cups chicken broth (low-sodium)
- 1 can (14 oz) diced tomatoes, undrained
- 1 teaspoon dried sage
- 1 teaspoon dried rosemary
- Salt and black pepper to taste
- Fresh parsley, chopped, for garnish

Directions:

1. In a large pot, heat olive oil over medium-high heat.

2. Add diced onion and minced garlic to the pot. Sauté until the onion is translucent.

3. Add ground turkey to the pot and cook until browned.

4. Stir in diced butternut squash and sliced carrots.

5. Pour in chicken broth and diced tomatoes with their juice.

6. Add dried sage and dried rosemary to the pot. Season with salt and black pepper to taste.

7. Bring the stew to a simmer and let it cook for about 25-30 minutes or until the vegetables are tender.

8. Adjust seasoning if needed.

9. Ladle the Turkey and Butternut Squash Stew into bowls.

10. Garnish with fresh chopped parsley before serving.

Chicken and Mushroom Barley Stew

Ingredients:

- 1.5 pounds boneless, skinless chicken thighs, cut into bite-sized pieces
- 2 tablespoons olive oil
- 1 onion, diced
- 2 carrots, sliced
- 2 celery stalks, sliced
- 8 ounces cremini mushrooms, sliced
- 1 cup pearl barley, rinsed

- 4 cups chicken broth (low-sodium)
- 1 teaspoon dried thyme
- 1 bay leaf
- Salt and black pepper to taste
- Fresh parsley, chopped, for garnish

Directions:

1. In a large pot, heat olive oil over medium-high heat.
2. Add diced onion, sliced carrots, and sliced celery to the pot. Sauté until the vegetables begin to soften.
3. Add chicken pieces to the pot and cook until browned.
4. Stir in sliced cremini mushrooms and cook until they release their moisture.
5. Add rinsed pearl barley, chicken broth, dried thyme, and bay leaf to the pot.
6. Season with salt and black pepper to taste.
7. Bring the stew to a simmer, then reduce the heat to low, cover, and let it cook for about 40-45 minutes or until the barley is tender.
8. Adjust seasoning if needed.
9. Ladle the Chicken and Mushroom Barley Stew into bowls.
10. Garnish with fresh chopped parsley before serving.

Spicy Lentil and Kale Soup

Ingredients:

- 1 cup dried green or brown lentils, rinsed
- 2 tablespoons olive oil
- 1 onion, diced
- 3 cloves garlic, minced
- 1 teaspoon ground cumin
- 1 teaspoon smoked paprika
- 1/2 teaspoon cayenne pepper (adjust to taste)
- 1 can (14 oz) diced tomatoes, undrained
- 6 cups vegetable broth (low-sodium)
- 1 bunch kale, stems removed and leaves chopped
- Salt and black pepper to taste
- Fresh lemon wedges, for serving

Directions:

1. In a large pot, heat olive oil over medium-high heat.
2. Add diced onion and minced garlic to the pot. Sauté until the onion is translucent.
3. Stir in ground cumin, smoked paprika, and cayenne pepper. Cook for an additional minute to release the spices' flavors.
4. Add rinsed lentils, diced tomatoes with their juice, and vegetable broth to the pot.

5. Bring the soup to a boil, then reduce the heat to low, cover, and let it simmer for about 20-25 minutes or until the lentils are tender.

6. Add chopped kale to the pot and simmer for an additional 5-7 minutes until the kale is wilted.

7. Season the soup with salt and black pepper to taste.

8. Ladle the Spicy Lentil and Kale Soup into bowls.

9. Serve with fresh lemon wedges for squeezing over the soup before enjoying.

Beef and Sweet Potato Stew

Ingredients:

- 1.5 pounds stew beef, cut into bite-sized pieces
- 2 tablespoons olive oil
- 1 onion, diced
- 3 cloves garlic, minced
- 2 sweet potatoes, peeled and diced
- 2 carrots, sliced
- 4 cups beef broth (low-sodium)
- 1 can (14 oz) crushed tomatoes
- 1 teaspoon dried thyme
- 1 teaspoon smoked paprika
- Salt and black pepper to taste
- Fresh parsley, chopped, for garnish

Directions:

1. In a large pot, heat olive oil over medium-high heat.
2. Add diced onion and minced garlic to the pot. Sauté until the onion is softened.
3. Add stew beef to the pot and brown on all sides.
4. Stir in diced sweet potatoes and sliced carrots.
5. Pour in beef broth and crushed tomatoes with their juice.
6. Add dried thyme and smoked paprika to the pot. Season with salt and black pepper to taste.
7. Bring the stew to a simmer, then reduce the heat to low, cover, and let it cook for about 45-50 minutes or until the beef is tender.
8. Adjust seasoning if needed.
9. Ladle the Beef and Sweet Potato Stew into bowls.
10. Garnish with fresh chopped parsley before serving.
11. Enjoy this hearty and nourishing Blood Type O Diet-friendly stew!

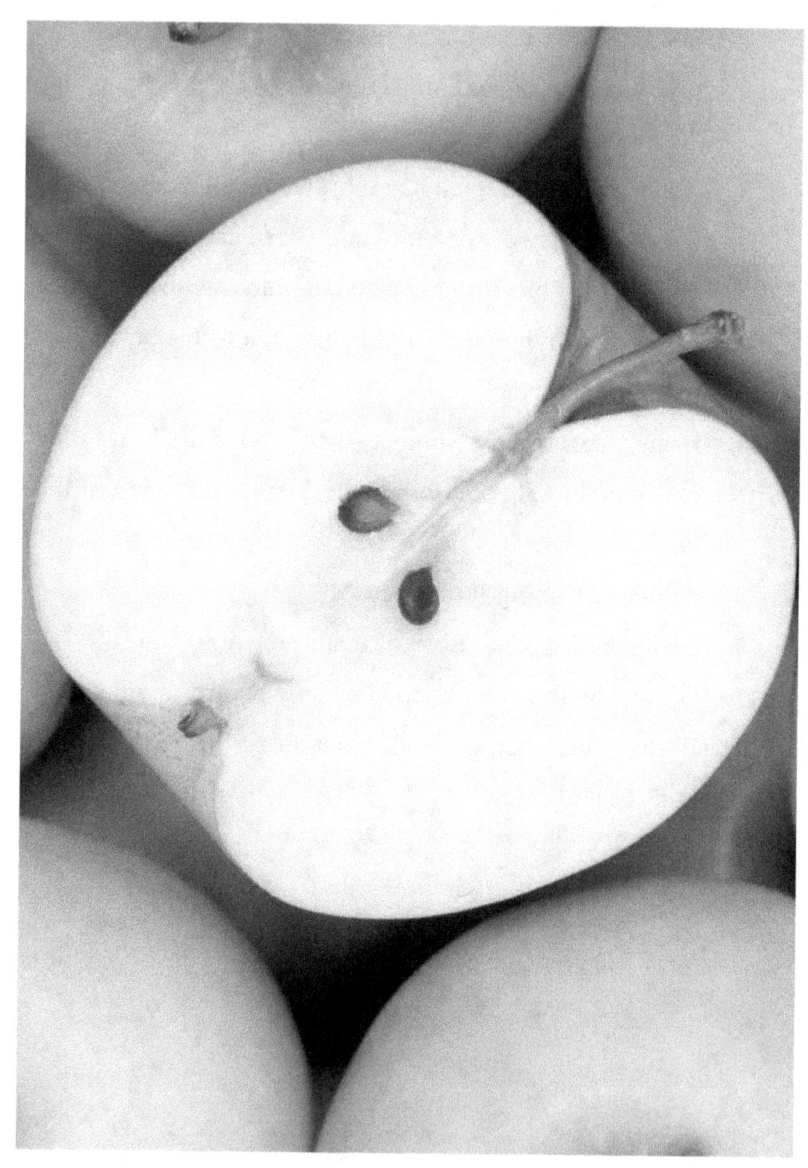

CHAPTER 8: FISH AND POULTRY DISHES

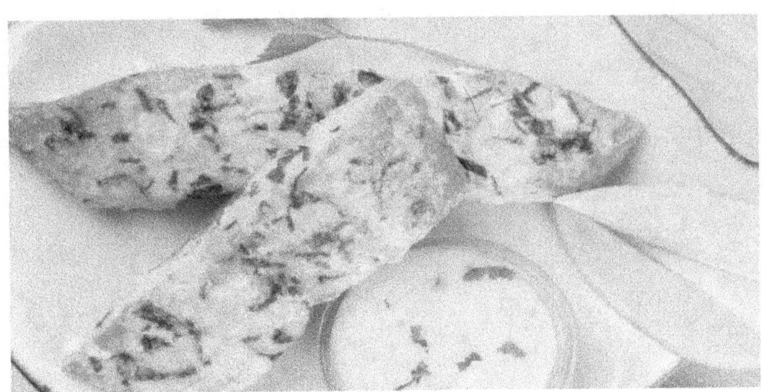

Baked Lemon Herb Salmon

Ingredients:

- 4 salmon filets
- 2 tablespoons olive oil
- 1 lemon, thinly sliced
- 2 cloves garlic, minced
- 1 teaspoon dried thyme
- 1 teaspoon dried rosemary
- Salt and black pepper to taste
- Fresh parsley, chopped, for garnish

Directions:

1. Preheat your oven to 400°F (200°C).

2. Place the salmon filets on a baking sheet lined with parchment paper.

3. In a small bowl, mix olive oil, minced garlic, dried thyme, dried rosemary, salt, and black pepper.

4. Brush the olive oil and herb mixture over each salmon filet, ensuring they are well coated.

5. Place lemon slices on top of each salmon filet.

6. Bake in the preheated oven for about 15-20 minutes or until the salmon is cooked through and flakes easily with a fork.

7. Garnish with fresh chopped parsley before serving.

8. Serve the Baked Lemon Herb Salmon with your favorite steamed vegetables or a side salad.

Grilled Herb Chicken Breast with Lemon

Ingredients:

- 4 boneless, skinless chicken breasts
- 2 tablespoons olive oil
- 2 teaspoons dried oregano
- 1 teaspoon dried thyme
- 1 teaspoon paprika
- Zest of 1 lemon
- Juice of 1 lemon
- 3 cloves garlic, minced

- Salt and black pepper to taste

- Fresh basil, chopped, for garnish

Directions:

1. Preheat your grill or grill pan to medium-high heat.

2. In a small bowl, combine olive oil, dried oregano, dried thyme, paprika, lemon zest, lemon juice, minced garlic, salt, and black pepper.

3. Brush the herb and lemon mixture over each chicken breast, ensuring they are well coated.

4. Place the chicken breasts on the preheated grill and cook for about 6-8 minutes per side or until the internal temperature reaches 165°F (74°C) and the chicken is no longer pink in the center.

5. Remove the grilled chicken from the heat and let it rest for a few minutes.

6. Garnish with fresh chopped basil before serving.

7. Serve the Grilled Herb Chicken Breast with a side of steamed vegetables or a crisp salad.

Rosemary Lemon Chicken Skewers

Ingredients:

- 1.5 pounds boneless, skinless chicken breasts, cut into bite-sized pieces

- 2 tablespoons olive oil

- Zest of 1 lemon

- Juice of 1 lemon

- 2 tablespoons fresh rosemary, finely chopped

- 3 cloves garlic, minced

- Salt and black pepper to taste

- Wooden skewers, soaked in water for 30 minutes

- Fresh parsley, chopped, for garnish

Directions:

1. In a bowl, combine olive oil, lemon zest, lemon juice, chopped rosemary, minced garlic, salt, and black pepper.

2. Add the bite-sized chicken pieces to the bowl and toss until well-coated. Let it marinate for at least 20 minutes.

3. Preheat your grill or grill pan to medium-high heat.

4. Thread the marinated chicken pieces onto the soaked wooden skewers.

5. Grill the chicken skewers for about 5-7 minutes per side or until fully cooked and nicely charred.

6. Remove the skewers from the grill and let them rest for a few minutes.

7. Garnish with fresh chopped parsley before serving.

8. Serve the Rosemary Lemon Chicken Skewers with a side of your favorite roasted vegetables or a crisp salad.

Garlic Ginger Turkey Stir-Fry

Ingredients:

- 1 pound ground turkey
- 2 tablespoons sesame oil
- 1 onion, thinly sliced
- 1 red bell pepper, thinly sliced
- 1 yellow bell pepper, thinly sliced
- 1 cup snap peas, ends trimmed
- 3 cloves garlic, minced
- 1 tablespoon fresh ginger, grated
- 3 tablespoons tamari or soy sauce (low-sodium)
- 1 tablespoon honey or maple syrup
- 1 teaspoon rice vinegar
- 1 teaspoon chili paste (optional, for heat)
- Sesame seeds (for garnish)
- Green onions, sliced (for garnish)
- Cooked quinoa or rice (optional, for serving)

Directions:

1. In a large skillet or wok, heat sesame oil over medium-high heat.
2. Add ground turkey to the skillet and cook until browned.
3. Add thinly sliced onion, red bell pepper, yellow bell pepper, and snap peas to the skillet. Stir-fry for 5-7 minutes or until the vegetables are tender-crisp.

4. Stir in minced garlic and grated ginger. Cook for an additional minute.

5. In a small bowl, mix tamari or soy sauce, honey or maple syrup, rice vinegar, and chili paste if using.

6. Pour the sauce mixture over the turkey and vegetables. Stir to combine and ensure everything is well-coated.

7. Cook for an additional 2-3 minutes until the flavors meld.

8. Garnish the stir-fry with sesame seeds and sliced green onions.

9. Serve the Garlic Ginger Turkey Stir-Fry over cooked quinoa or rice if preferred.

Baked Dijon Herb Tilapia

Ingredients:

- 4 tilapia filets
- 2 tablespoons Dijon mustard
- 2 tablespoons olive oil
- 1 tablespoon fresh dill, chopped
- 1 tablespoon fresh parsley, chopped
- 1 teaspoon lemon juice
- 2 cloves garlic, minced
- Salt and black pepper to taste
- Lemon wedges (for serving)

Directions:

1. Preheat your oven to 400°F (200°C).

2. In a small bowl, whisk together Dijon mustard, olive oil, chopped dill, chopped parsley, lemon juice, minced garlic, salt, and black pepper.

3. Place the tilapia filets on a baking sheet lined with parchment paper.

4. Brush the Dijon herb mixture over each tilapia filet, ensuring they are well coated.

5. Bake in the preheated oven for about 12-15 minutes or until the tilapia is cooked through and flakes easily with a fork.

6. Remove from the oven and let it rest for a couple of minutes.

7. Serve the Baked Dijon Herb Tilapia with lemon wedges on the side.

Lemon Garlic Butter Salmon Packets

Ingredients:

- 4 salmon filets
- 4 tablespoons unsalted butter, melted
- 2 tablespoons fresh lemon juice
- 3 cloves garlic, minced
- 1 teaspoon dried thyme

- 1 teaspoon paprika

- Salt and black pepper to taste

- Lemon slices (for garnish)

- Fresh parsley, chopped (for garnish)

Directions:

1. Preheat your oven to 400°F (200°C).

2. Place each salmon filet on a piece of parchment paper or aluminum foil.

3. In a bowl, mix melted butter, fresh lemon juice, minced garlic, dried thyme, paprika, salt, and black pepper.

4. Spoon the lemon garlic butter mixture over each salmon filet, ensuring they are well coated.

5. Fold the parchment paper or aluminum foil over the salmon to create packets, sealing the edges.

6. Place the packets on a baking sheet and bake in the preheated oven for about 15-18 minutes or until the salmon is cooked through.

7. Carefully open the packets, garnish with lemon slices and chopped fresh parsley.

8. Serve the Lemon Garlic Butter Salmon with your favorite steamed vegetables or a side salad.

Lemon Herb Chicken Thighs

Ingredients:

- 4 bone-in, skin-on chicken thighs
- 2 tablespoons olive oil
- Zest of 1 lemon
- Juice of 1 lemon
- 2 tablespoons fresh rosemary, chopped
- 3 cloves garlic, minced
- Salt and black pepper to taste
- Lemon slices (for garnish)
- Fresh thyme, for garnish

Directions:

1. Preheat your oven to 400°F (200°C).
2. In a bowl, mix olive oil, lemon zest, lemon juice, chopped rosemary, minced garlic, salt, and black pepper.
3. Pat the chicken thighs dry with paper towels and place them in a baking dish.
4. Brush the lemon herb mixture over each chicken thigh, ensuring they are well coated.
5. Arrange lemon slices on top of each chicken thigh for extra flavor.
6. Bake in the preheated oven for about 30-35 minutes or until the chicken is cooked through, and the skin is golden and crispy.

7. Remove from the oven and let it rest for a few minutes.

8. Garnish with fresh thyme before serving.

9. Serve the Lemon Herb Chicken Thighs with your preferred roasted vegetables or a side of quinoa.

Balsamic Honey Glazed Chicken Breasts

Ingredients:

- 4 boneless, skinless chicken breasts
- 1/4 cup balsamic vinegar
- 2 tablespoons honey
- 2 tablespoons olive oil
- 2 cloves garlic, minced
- 1 teaspoon dried thyme
- Salt and black pepper to taste
- Fresh basil, chopped (for garnish)

Directions:

1. Preheat your oven to 400°F (200°C).

2. In a small bowl, whisk together balsamic vinegar, honey, olive oil, minced garlic, dried thyme, salt, and black pepper.

3. Place the chicken breasts in a baking dish.

4. Pour the balsamic honey mixture over the chicken breasts, making sure they are well coated.

5. Bake in the preheated oven for about 20-25 minutes or until the chicken is cooked through and juices run clear.

6. Baste the chicken with the glaze from the pan halfway through cooking.

7. Remove from the oven and let it rest for a few minutes.

8. Garnish with fresh chopped basil before serving.

9. Serve the Balsamic Honey Glazed Chicken Breasts with a side of steamed broccoli or your favorite greens.

Coconut Lime Baked Cod

Ingredients:

- 4 cod filets
- 1/2 cup coconut milk
- Zest and juice of 2 limes
- 2 tablespoons coconut oil, melted
- 2 teaspoons ground coriander
- 1 teaspoon ground cumin
- 2 cloves garlic, minced
- Salt and black pepper to taste
- Fresh cilantro, chopped (for garnish)
- Lime wedges (for serving)

Directions:

1. Preheat your oven to 400°F (200°C).

2. In a bowl, combine coconut milk, lime zest, lime juice, melted coconut oil, ground coriander, ground cumin, minced garlic, salt, and black pepper.

3. Place the cod filets in a baking dish.

4. Pour the coconut lime mixture over the cod filets, ensuring they are well coated.

5. Bake in the preheated oven for about 15-20 minutes or until the cod is opaque and flakes easily with a fork.

6. Remove from the oven and let it rest for a few minutes.

7. Garnish with fresh chopped cilantro.

8. Serve the Coconut Lime Baked Cod with lime wedges on the side.

Herb-Crusted Baked Salmon

Ingredients:

- 4 salmon filets
- 2 tablespoons Dijon mustard
- 2 tablespoons olive oil
- 1 tablespoon fresh dill, chopped
- 1 tablespoon fresh parsley, chopped
- 1 teaspoon lemon zest
- 2 cloves garlic, minced
- Salt and black pepper to taste
- Almond flour (or breadcrumbs) for coating

Directions:

1. Preheat your oven to 400°F (200°C).
2. In a bowl, mix Dijon mustard, olive oil, chopped dill, chopped parsley, lemon zest, minced garlic, salt, and black pepper.
3. Pat the salmon filets dry with paper towels.
4. Coat each salmon filet with the Dijon herb mixture.
5. Roll each salmon filet in almond flour or breadcrumbs to create a light crust.
6. Place the coated salmon filets on a baking sheet lined with parchment paper.
7. Bake in the preheated oven for about 12-15 minutes or until the salmon is cooked through and the crust is golden.
8. Remove from the oven and let it rest for a couple of minutes.
9. Serve the Herb-Crusted Baked Salmon with a side of steamed vegetables or a crisp salad.

Mango Chipotle Grilled Chicken

Ingredients:

- 4 boneless, skinless chicken breasts
- 1 ripe mango, peeled and diced
- 2 tablespoons olive oil

- 2 tablespoons chipotle peppers in adobo sauce, minced
- 1 tablespoon lime juice
- 1 teaspoon ground cumin
- 2 cloves garlic, minced
- Salt and black pepper to taste
- Fresh cilantro, chopped (for garnish)

Directions:

1. In a blender or food processor, combine diced mango, olive oil, minced chipotle peppers, lime juice, ground cumin, minced garlic, salt, and black pepper. Blend until smooth.

2. Place the chicken breasts in a shallow dish and coat them with the mango chipotle marinade. Allow them to marinate for at least 30 minutes.

3. Preheat your grill or grill pan to medium-high heat.

4. Grill the marinated chicken breasts for about 6-8 minutes per side or until fully cooked and grill marks appear.

5. Remove from the grill and let them rest for a few minutes.

6. Garnish with freshly chopped cilantro.

7. Serve the Mango Chipotle Grilled Chicken with a side of quinoa or your favorite roasted vegetables.

Pesto Baked Trout

Ingredients:

- 4 trout filets
- 1 cup fresh basil leaves
- 1/4 cup pine nuts
- 2 cloves garlic, minced
- 1/2 cup Parmesan cheese, grated
- 1/3 cup olive oil
- Juice of 1 lemon
- Salt and black pepper to taste
- Lemon wedges (for serving)
- Fresh parsley, chopped (for garnish)

Directions:

1. Preheat your oven to 400°F (200°C).
2. In a food processor, combine fresh basil, pine nuts, minced garlic, grated Parmesan cheese, olive oil, and lemon juice. Blend until you have a smooth pesto sauce.
3. Season the trout filets with salt and black pepper.
4. Place the trout filets on a baking sheet lined with parchment paper.
5. Spread a generous layer of the pesto sauce over each trout filet, covering them evenly.
6. Bake in the preheated oven for about 15-20 minutes or until the trout is cooked through and flakes easily.

7. Remove from the oven and let it rest for a couple of minutes.

8. Garnish with chopped fresh parsley and serve with lemon wedges on the side.

9. Enjoy this flavorful and easy-to-make Blood Type O Diet-friendly fish dish!

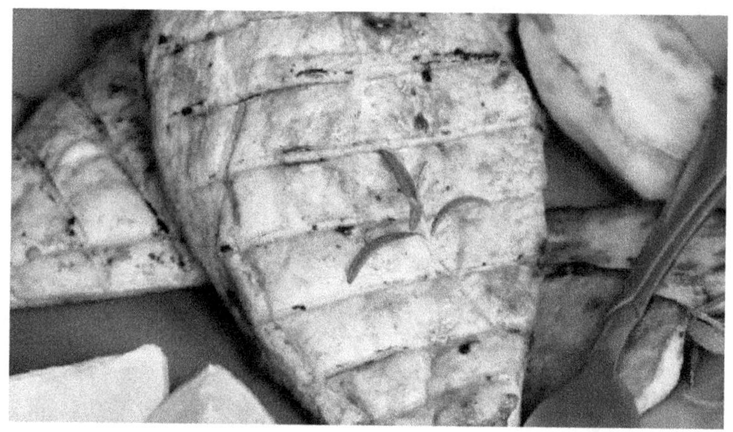

CHAPTER 9: VEGETABLE DISHES

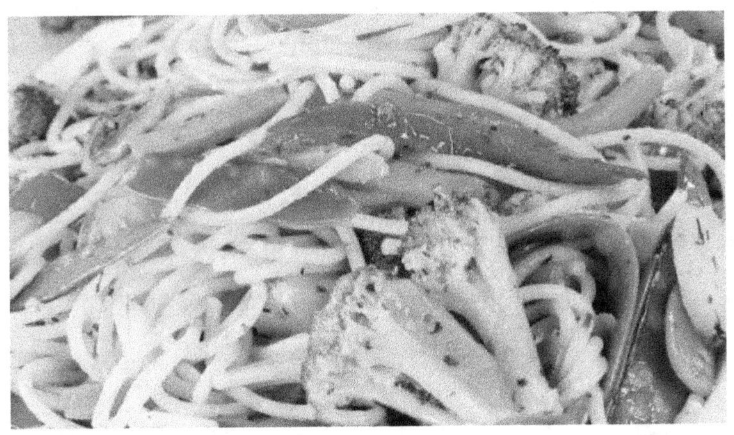

Roasted Asparagus with Lemon and Parmesan

Ingredients:

- 1 bunch asparagus, tough ends trimmed
- 2 tablespoons olive oil
- Zest of 1 lemon
- 2 tablespoons freshly squeezed lemon juice
- 1/4 cup grated Parmesan cheese
- Salt and black pepper to taste

Directions:

1. Preheat your oven to 400°F (200°C).
2. Place trimmed asparagus on a baking sheet.

3. Drizzle olive oil over the asparagus and toss to coat evenly.

4. Sprinkle lemon zest and lemon juice over the asparagus.

5. Season with salt and black pepper to taste, then toss again to ensure even coating.

6. Roast in the preheated oven for about 12-15 minutes, or until the asparagus is tender-crisp.

7. Remove from the oven and transfer to a serving platter.

8. Sprinkle grated Parmesan cheese over the roasted asparagus.

9. Serve and enjoy the Roasted Asparagus with Lemon and Parmesan.

Mushroom and Spinach Sauté with Garlic

Ingredients:

- 8 ounces mushrooms, sliced
- 4 cups fresh spinach leaves, washed
- 3 cloves garlic, minced
- 2 tablespoons olive oil
- 1 tablespoon balsamic vinegar
- Salt and black pepper to taste
- Crushed red pepper flakes (optional, for heat)

Directions:

1. In a large skillet, heat olive oil over medium heat.

2. Add sliced mushrooms to the skillet and sauté until they release their moisture and become golden brown.

3. Stir in minced garlic and continue to sauté for an additional minute until fragrant.

4. Add fresh spinach to the skillet and toss until wilted.

5. Drizzle balsamic vinegar over the mushrooms and spinach. Stir to combine.

6. Season with salt and black pepper to taste. Add crushed red pepper flakes if you prefer some heat.

7. Continue to cook for 2-3 minutes until the flavors meld together.

8. Transfer the Mushroom and Spinach Sauté with Garlic to a serving dish.

9. Serve this delightful and easy-to-make Blood Type O Diet-friendly vegetable dish.

Grilled Eggplant with Tahini Dressing

Ingredients:

- 1 large eggplant, sliced into rounds
- 3 tablespoons olive oil
- 2 tablespoons tahini
- 1 tablespoon lemon juice
- 2 cloves garlic, minced
- 1 teaspoon ground cumin

- Salt and black pepper to taste
- Fresh parsley, chopped (for garnish)

Directions:

1. Preheat your grill or grill pan over medium-high heat.
2. Brush both sides of eggplant slices with olive oil.
3. Grill the eggplant slices for 4-5 minutes on each side or until they are tender and have nice grill marks.
4. In a small bowl, whisk together tahini, lemon juice, minced garlic, ground cumin, salt, and black pepper.
5. Arrange the grilled eggplant slices on a serving platter.
6. Drizzle the tahini dressing over the eggplant slices.
7. Garnish with fresh chopped parsley.
8. Serve and enjoy the Grilled Eggplant with Tahini Dressing.

Sweet Potato and Kale Hash

Ingredients:

- 2 medium sweet potatoes, peeled and diced
- 2 cups kale, stems removed and chopped
- 1 red onion, finely chopped
- 2 tablespoons olive oil
- 1 teaspoon smoked paprika
- 1/2 teaspoon cumin
- Salt and black pepper to taste

- Poached or fried eggs (optional, for serving)

Directions:

1. In a large skillet, heat olive oil over medium heat.

2. Add chopped red onion to the skillet and sauté until translucent.

3. Add diced sweet potatoes to the skillet and cook for 8-10 minutes or until they are tender and slightly crispy.

4. Sprinkle smoked paprika and cumin over the sweet potatoes. Stir to combine.

5. Add chopped kale to the skillet and cook until wilted.

6. Season with salt and black pepper to taste. Adjust the seasoning as needed.

7. Continue to cook for an additional 3-5 minutes until the flavors meld together.

8. Serve the Sweet Potato and Kale Hash on a plate, optionally topped with poached or fried eggs.

Zesty Broccoli and Bell Pepper Stir-Fry

Ingredients:

- 2 cups broccoli florets
- 1 red bell pepper, thinly sliced
- 1 yellow bell pepper, thinly sliced
- 2 tablespoons olive oil

- 2 tablespoons soy sauce (or tamari for a gluten-free option)
- 1 tablespoon rice vinegar
- 1 teaspoon honey
- 2 cloves garlic, minced
- 1 teaspoon fresh ginger, grated
- Sesame seeds (for garnish)
- Green onions, sliced (for garnish)

Directions:

1. In a large wok or skillet, heat olive oil over medium-high heat.
2. Add minced garlic and grated ginger, stir-frying for about 30 seconds until fragrant.
3. Add broccoli florets and sliced bell peppers to the wok. Stir-fry for 3-4 minutes until the vegetables are tender-crisp.
4. In a small bowl, whisk together soy sauce, rice vinegar, and honey.
5. Pour the sauce over the vegetables and toss to coat evenly. Cook for an additional 1-2 minutes.
6. Transfer the Zesty Broccoli and Bell Pepper Stir-Fry to a serving dish.
7. Garnish with sesame seeds and sliced green onions.

Spaghetti Squash Primavera

Ingredients:

- 1 medium-sized spaghetti squash
- 2 tablespoons olive oil
- 1 cup cherry tomatoes, halved
- 1 zucchini, thinly sliced
- 1 yellow bell pepper, julienned
- 2 cloves garlic, minced
- 1/4 cup fresh basil, chopped
- Salt and black pepper to taste
- Grated Parmesan cheese (optional, for garnish)

Directions:

1. Preheat your oven to 400°F (200°C).
2. Cut the spaghetti squash in half lengthwise, scoop out the seeds, and place the halves on a baking sheet.
3. Drizzle each half with 1 tablespoon of olive oil, then season with salt and black pepper.
4. Roast in the preheated oven for 40-45 minutes or until the flesh easily shreds into spaghetti-like strands with a fork.
5. While the squash is roasting, heat the remaining olive oil in a large skillet over medium heat.
6. Add minced garlic and sauté until fragrant, about 1 minute.

7. Add cherry tomatoes, zucchini, and yellow bell pepper to the skillet. Cook for 5-7 minutes until the vegetables are tender-crisp.

8. Once the spaghetti squash is done, use a fork to scrape out the strands and add them to the skillet with the sautéed vegetables.

9. Toss everything together until well combined. Stir in fresh basil.

10. Adjust seasoning with salt and black pepper to taste.

11. Serve this Spaghetti Squash Primavera with optional grated Parmesan cheese and enjoy!

Cauliflower and Chickpea Curry

Ingredients:

- 1 small cauliflower, cut into florets
- 1 can (15 oz) chickpeas, drained and rinsed
- 1 onion, finely chopped
- 2 tomatoes, chopped
- 2 cloves garlic, minced
- 1 tablespoon ginger, grated
- 1 can (14 oz) coconut milk
- 2 tablespoons curry powder
- 1 teaspoon turmeric
- 1 teaspoon cumin

- 1/2 teaspoon cayenne pepper (adjust to taste)
- Salt and black pepper to taste
- Fresh cilantro, chopped (for garnish)
- Cooked brown rice (for serving)

Directions:

1. In a large skillet or pot, sauté chopped onion, garlic, and ginger until softened.
2. Add cauliflower florets and cook for 3-5 minutes until slightly browned.
3. Stir in curry powder, turmeric, cumin, and cayenne pepper. Cook for an additional 1-2 minutes until fragrant.
4. Add chopped tomatoes and cook until they start to break down.
5. Pour in coconut milk, stirring to combine. Bring the mixture to a simmer.
6. Add chickpeas to the curry and let it simmer for 15-20 minutes, or until the cauliflower is tender.
7. Season with salt and black pepper to taste.
8. Serve the Cauliflower and Chickpea Curry over cooked brown rice.
9. Garnish with fresh cilantro.

Stir-Fried Asparagus with Almonds

Ingredients:

- 1 bunch asparagus, trimmed and cut into bite-sized pieces
- 2 tablespoons sesame oil
- 1/4 cup sliced almonds
- 2 cloves garlic, minced
- 1 tablespoon soy sauce (or tamari for a gluten-free option)
- 1 teaspoon rice vinegar
- 1 teaspoon honey
- Sesame seeds (for garnish)
- Green onions, sliced (for garnish)

Directions:

1. Heat sesame oil in a large skillet or wok over medium-high heat.
2. Add sliced almonds to the skillet and stir-fry for 1-2 minutes until they are lightly toasted. Remove almonds and set them aside.
3. In the same skillet, add minced garlic and stir-fry for about 30 seconds until fragrant.
4. Add asparagus pieces to the skillet and stir-fry for 3-5 minutes until they are tender-crisp.

5. In a small bowl, whisk together soy sauce, rice vinegar, and honey.

6. Pour the sauce over the asparagus and toss to coat evenly. Cook for an additional 1-2 minutes.

7. Sprinkle the toasted almonds over the stir-fried asparagus.

8. Garnish with sesame seeds and sliced green onions.

9. Serve this Stir-Fried Asparagus with Almonds as a flavorful vegetable dish.

Turmeric Roasted Carrots

Ingredients:

- 1 pound carrots, peeled and cut into sticks
- 2 tablespoons olive oil
- 1 teaspoon ground turmeric
- 1 teaspoon ground cumin
- 1/2 teaspoon paprika
- Salt and black pepper to taste
- Fresh cilantro, chopped (for garnish)

Directions:

1. Preheat your oven to 400°F (200°C).

2. In a large bowl, toss the carrot sticks with olive oil, ground turmeric, ground cumin, paprika, salt, and black pepper until well coated.

3. Spread the seasoned carrots in a single layer on a baking sheet.

4. Roast in the preheated oven for 20-25 minutes or until the carrots are tender and slightly caramelized.

5. Once done, transfer the Turmeric Roasted Carrots to a serving platter.

6. Garnish with fresh chopped cilantro for a burst of herbaceous flavor.

7. Serve these flavorful Turmeric Roasted Carrots as a colorful and easy-to-make Blood Type O Diet-friendly vegetable dish.

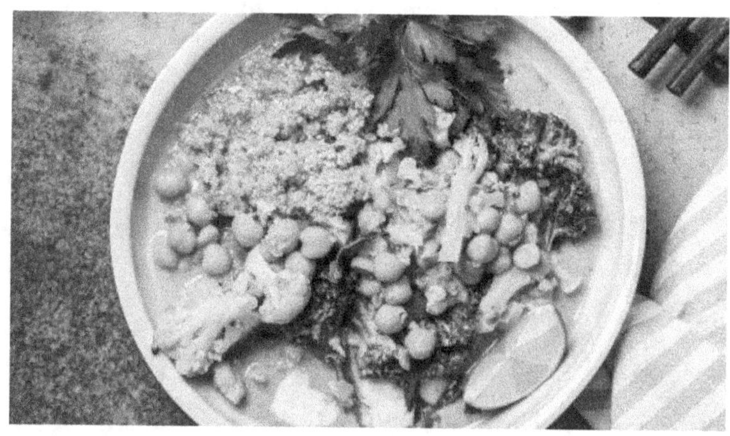

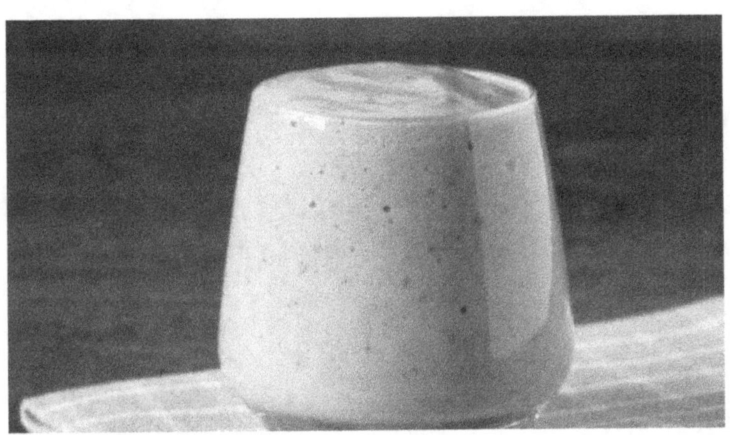

Berry Green Smoothie

Ingredients:

- 1 cup spinach leaves, washed
- 1/2 cup blueberries, fresh or frozen
- 1/2 cup strawberries, hulled and halved
- 1/2 banana
- 1 tablespoon chia seeds
- 1 cup almond milk (or any Blood Type O-friendly alternative)
- Ice cubes (optional)

Directions:

1. In a blender, combine spinach, blueberries, strawberries, banana, chia seeds, and almond milk.

2. Blend on high speed until the mixture is smooth and creamy.

3. If you prefer a colder smoothie, add ice cubes and blend again until well combined.

4. Pour the Berry Green Smoothie into a glass.

5. Optionally, garnish with a few whole berries or a sprinkle of chia seeds for added texture.

Tropical Green Smoothie

Ingredients:

- 1 cup kale, washed and stems removed
- 1/2 cup pineapple chunks, fresh or frozen
- 1/2 cup mango chunks, fresh or frozen
- 1/2 banana
- 1 tablespoon flaxseeds
- 1 cup coconut water (or any Blood Type O-friendly liquid)
- Ice cubes (optional)

Directions:

1. In a blender, combine kale, pineapple chunks, mango chunks, banana, flaxseeds, and coconut water.

2. Blend on high speed until the mixture is smooth and creamy.

3. If you like a colder smoothie, add ice cubes and blend again until well combined.

4. Pour the Tropical Green Smoothie into a glass.

5. Optionally, garnish with a slice of pineapple or a sprinkle of flaxseeds for extra flair.

Citrus Berry Blast Smoothie

Ingredients:

- 1 cup kale, washed and stems removed
- 1/2 cup mixed berries (blueberries, raspberries, or strawberries), fresh or frozen
- 1/2 orange, peeled and segmented
- 1/2 banana
- 1 tablespoon pumpkin seeds
- 1 cup water or Blood Type O-friendly juice (like cherry or cranberry)
- Ice cubes (optional)

Directions:

1. In a blender, combine kale, mixed berries, orange segments, banana, pumpkin seeds, and water or Blood Type O-friendly juice.

2. Blend on high speed until the mixture is smooth and vibrant.

3. If you prefer a colder smoothie, add ice cubes and blend again until well combined.

4. Pour the Citrus Berry Blast Smoothie into a glass.

5. Optionally, garnish with a slice of orange or a sprinkle of pumpkin seeds for added texture.

Peachy Green Energizer Smoothie

Ingredients:

- 1 cup spinach leaves, washed
- 1 cup sliced peaches, fresh or frozen
- 1/2 banana
- 1 tablespoon almond butter
- 1 teaspoon honey (optional)
- 1 cup water or Blood Type O-friendly liquid
- Ice cubes (optional)

Directions:

1. In a blender, combine spinach, sliced peaches, banana, almond butter, honey (if using), and water or Blood Type O-friendly liquid.

2. Blend on high speed until the mixture is smooth and velvety.

3. Add ice cubes if you desire a chilled smoothie, then blend again until well combined.

4. Pour the Peachy Green Energizer Smoothie into a glass.

5. Optionally, garnish with a slice of peach or a drizzle of
   almond butter for extra flavor.

Minty Blueberry Bliss Smoothie

Ingredients:

- 1 cup kale, washed and stems removed
- 1/2 cup blueberries, fresh or frozen
- 1/2 avocado, peeled and pitted
- 1 tablespoon fresh mint leaves
- 1 tablespoon chia seeds
- 1 cup coconut water (or any Blood Type O-friendly liquid)
- Ice cubes (optional)

Directions:

1. In a blender, combine kale, blueberries, avocado, fresh mint leaves, chia seeds, and coconut water.
2. Blend on high speed until the mixture is smooth and vibrant.
3. If you prefer a colder smoothie, add ice cubes and blend again until well combined.
4. Pour the Minty Blueberry Bliss Smoothie into a glass.
5. Optionally, garnish with a sprig of fresh mint or a few whole blueberries for a burst of color.

Tangy Mango Turmeric Smoothie

Ingredients:

- 1 cup spinach leaves, washed
- 1/2 cup diced mango, fresh or frozen
- 1/2 banana
- 1/2 teaspoon turmeric powder
- 1 tablespoon hemp seeds
- 1 cup pomegranate juice (or any Blood Type O-friendly liquid)
- Ice cubes (optional)

Directions:

1. In a blender, combine spinach, diced mango, banana, turmeric powder, hemp seeds, and pomegranate juice.
2. Blend on high speed until the mixture is smooth and vibrant.
3. If you enjoy a colder smoothie, add ice cubes and blend again until well combined.
4. Pour the Tangy Mango Turmeric Smoothie into a glass.
5. Optionally, garnish with a slice of mango or a sprinkle of hemp seeds for added texture.

Berry Beet Burst Smoothie

Ingredients:

- 1 cup beet slices, cooked and cooled
- 1/2 cup mixed berries (strawberries, raspberries, or blueberries), fresh or frozen
- 1/2 banana
- 1 tablespoon ground flaxseeds
- 1 cup water or Blood Type O-friendly juice (like cherry or cranberry)
- Ice cubes (optional)

Directions:

1. In a blender, combine beet slices, mixed berries, banana, ground flaxseeds, and water or Blood Type O-friendly juice.
2. Blend on high speed until the mixture is smooth and vibrant.
3. Add ice cubes if you prefer a colder smoothie, then blend again until well combined.
4. Pour the Berry Beet Burst Smoothie into a glass.
5. Optionally, garnish with a few whole berries or a sprinkle of flaxseeds for added visual appeal.

Pineapple Ginger Zing Smoothie

Ingredients:

- 1 cup kale, washed and stems removed
- 1/2 cup pineapple chunks, fresh or frozen
- 1/2 banana
- 1 tablespoon grated fresh ginger
- 1 tablespoon sunflower seeds
- 1 cup coconut water (or any Blood Type O-friendly liquid)
- Ice cubes (optional)

Directions:

1. In a blender, combine kale, pineapple chunks, banana, grated ginger, sunflower seeds, and coconut water.
2. Blend on high speed until the mixture is smooth and invigorating.
3. If you prefer a colder smoothie, add ice cubes and blend again until well combined.
4. Pour the Pineapple Ginger Zing Smoothie into a glass.
5. Optionally, garnish with a slice of pineapple or a sprinkle of sunflower seeds for extra texture.

Citrus Minty Greens Smoothie

Ingredients:

- 1 cup spinach leaves, washed
- 1/2 orange, peeled and segmented
- 1/2 kiwi, peeled and sliced
- 1/2 banana
- 1 tablespoon fresh mint leaves
- 1 tablespoon chia seeds
- 1 cup green tea (cooled) or any Blood Type O-friendly liquid
- Ice cubes (optional)

Directions:

1. In a blender, combine spinach leaves, orange segments, kiwi slices, banana, fresh mint leaves, chia seeds, and green tea or Blood Type O-friendly liquid.
2. Blend on high speed until the mixture is smooth and citrusy.
3. If you prefer a colder smoothie, add ice cubes and blend again until well combined.
4. Pour the Citrus Minty Greens Smoothie into a glass.
5. Optionally, garnish with a sprig of fresh mint or a slice of orange for a burst of flavor.

Apple Cinnamon Crunch Smoothie

Ingredients:

- 1 cup kale, washed and stems removed
- 1 medium apple, cored and chopped
- 1/2 banana
- 1 tablespoon almond butter
- 1/2 teaspoon ground cinnamon
- 1 cup almond milk (or any Blood Type O-friendly liquid)
- Ice cubes (optional)

Directions:

1. In a blender, combine kale, chopped apple, banana, almond butter, ground cinnamon, and almond milk.
2. Blend on high speed until the mixture is smooth and has a hint of apple-cinnamon goodness.
3. If you prefer a colder smoothie, add ice cubes and blend again until well combined.
4. Pour the Apple Cinnamon Crunch Smoothie into a glass.
5. Optionally, sprinkle a pinch of cinnamon on top or garnish with a few apple slices for added crunch.

Mango Avocado Bliss Smoothie

Ingredients:

- 1/2 cup spinach leaves, washed
- 1/2 cup diced mango, fresh or frozen
- 1/4 avocado, peeled and pitted
- 1/2 banana
- 1 tablespoon pumpkin seeds
- 1 cup coconut water (or any Blood Type O-friendly liquid)
- Ice cubes (optional)

Directions:

1. In a blender, combine spinach leaves, diced mango, avocado, banana, pumpkin seeds, and coconut water.
2. Blend on high speed until the mixture is smooth and has a creamy texture.
3. If you prefer a colder smoothie, add ice cubes and blend again until well combined.
4. Pour the Mango Avocado Bliss Smoothie into a glass.
5. Optionally, sprinkle some pumpkin seeds on top or garnish with a slice of mango for added sweetness.
6. Enjoy this tropical and nutrient-packed smoothie as a delicious addition to your Blood Type O Diet.

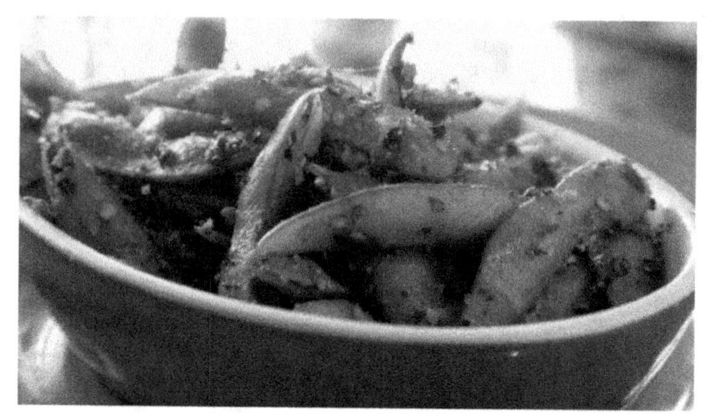

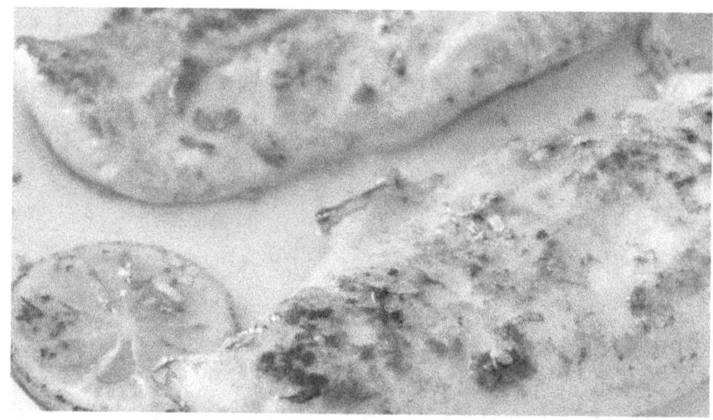

CONCLUSION

In conclusion, the "Blood Type O Diet Cookbook: Healthy Flavorful Recipes Tailored to Your Type O for Optimal Health and Wellness" provides a thorough and practical guide to aligning your dietary choices with the distinct qualities of Blood Type O. This cookbook not only offers a variety of tasty dishes, but it also encourages a holistic approach to health and fitness.

By implementing the Blood Type O Diet concepts into your culinary repertoire, you will begin on a path to improve your overall health. The meticulously created dishes stress lean meats, nutritious vegetables, and fruits, all of which are customized to Blood Type O's unique nutritional requirements. This method is intended to aid with weight control, increase energy levels, and maybe solve digestive issues.

What distinguishes this cookbook is its commitment to crafting meals that not only follow the Blood Type O Diet recommendations, but also celebrate the joy of eating. The meals are not only healthy, but also tasty, demonstrating that a blood type-specific diet can be both nutritious and fun.

By adopting the "Blood Type O Diet Cookbook," you are taking a proactive step toward a lifestyle that is compatible with your particular biology. May these recipes encourage you to enjoy the road of achieving health and wellbeing, one tasty and blood type-friendly meal at a time.

Happy Cooking!

Weekly
Meal Plan

Week: _______________

	BREAKFAST	LUNCH	DINNER	SNACKS
MON				
TUE				
WED				
THU				
FRI				
SAT				
SUN				

Shopping list

_______________ _______________

_______________ _______________

_______________ _______________

Notes:

Weekly
Meal Plan

Week: ___________

	BREAKFAST	LUNCH	DINNER	SNACKS
MON				
TUE				
WED				
THU				
FRI				
SAT				
SUN				

Shopping list

___________ ___________

___________ ___________

___________ ___________

Notes:

Weekly
Meal Plan

Week: ___________

	BREAKFAST	LUNCH	DINNER	SNACKS
MON				
TUE				
WED				
THU				
FRI				
SAT				
SUN				

Shopping list

______________   ______________

______________   ______________

______________   ______________

Notes:

Weekly
Meal Plan

Week: _______________

	BREAKFAST	LUNCH	DINNER	SNACKS
MON				
TUE				
WED				
THU				
FRI				
SAT				
SUN				

Shopping list

_______________ _______________

_______________ _______________

_______________ _______________

Notes:

Weekly
Meal Plan   Week: ___________

	BREAKFAST	LUNCH	DINNER	SNACKS
MON				
TUE				
WED				
THU				
FRI				
SAT				
SUN				

Shopping list

_______________   _______________

_______________   _______________

_______________   _______________

Notes:

Weekly
Meal Plan

Week: _______________

	BREAKFAST	LUNCH	DINNER	SNACKS
MON				
TUE				
WED				
THU				
FRI				
SAT				
SUN				

Shopping list

___________________ ___________________

___________________ ___________________

___________________ ___________________

Notes:

Weekly
Meal Plan

Week: ______________

	BREAKFAST	LUNCH	DINNER	SNACKS
MON				
TUE				
WED				
THU				
FRI				
SAT				
SUN				

Shopping list

______________   ______________

______________   ______________

____

Notes:

Weekly
Meal Plan

Week: _______________

	BREAKFAST	LUNCH	DINNER	SNACKS
MON				
TUE				
WED				
THU				
FRI				
SAT				
SUN				

Shopping list

_______________ _______________

_______________ _______________

_______________ _______________

Notes:

Weekly
Meal Plan

Week: _______________

	BREAKFAST	LUNCH	DINNER	SNACKS
MON				
TUE				
WED				
THU				
FRI				
SAT				
SUN				

Shopping list

_______________   _______________

_______________   _______________

_______________   _______________

Notes:

Weekly
Meal Plan

Week: ___________

	BREAKFAST	LUNCH	DINNER	SNACKS
MON				
TUE				
WED				
THU				
FRI				
SAT				
SUN				

Shopping list

_______________   _______________

_______________   _______________

_______________   _______________

Notes: